Standards for Blood Banks and Transfusion Services

29th Edition

Effective April 1, 2014

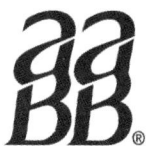

AABB
8101 Glenbrook Road
Bethesda, Maryland 20814-2749
United States of America

ISBN 978-1-56395-887-8
Printed in the United States

29th EDITION BLOOD BANK/TRANSFUSION SERVICE STANDARDS PROGRAM UNIT

Committee Members
Judith Levitt, MT(ASCP)SBB, Chair
Maureen A. Beaton, MT(ASCP)BB, CQA(ASQ)
Kaaron Benson, MD
Robert W. Braun, BS, MT(ASCP)SBB
Paula L. Brown, BS, MT(ASCP), JD
Dale E. Hammerschmidt, MD
Sarah J. Ilstrup, MD
Ronald E. Domen, MD
Sally Rudmann, PhD, MT(ASCP)SBB
Judy B. Smith, DM, MBA, MT(ASCP)SBB, CQM/OE(ASQ), CQA(ASQ)
Linda Stefaniak, BS, MT(ASCP)SBB, CQA(ASQ)CQM/OE
Christine Terranova, MT(ASCP)
Mary Townsend, MD

Liaisons Representing Other AABB Committees
Accreditation Program Committee, Donor Center Accreditation Program Unit—
    Susan M. Wilson, BS, MT(ASCP)SBB
Accreditation Program Committee, Transfusion Services Accreditation Program Unit—
    Sheryl Goertzen, MT(ASCP)BB, CLS
Information Systems Committee—Jeffrey Seok-Woo Jhang, MD
Transfusion-Transmitted Disease Committee—Debra A. Kessler, RN, MS
Uniform Donor History Questionnaire—Susan N. Rossman, MD, PhD

Representatives from Other Organizations
American Association of Tissue Banks—Scott Brubaker, CTBS
American College of Obstetricians and Gynecologists—George Saade, MD
American Heart Association—Neil Zakai, MD, MSc
American Red Cross—Anne F. Eder, MD, PhD
American Society for Apheresis—Nicholas Bandarenko, MD
Armed Services Blood Program Office (DoD)—Col. Richard Gonzales
Canadian Blood Services—Jennifer Biemans, BSc, ART; Beverly Padget, MT(ASCP), CQA(ASQ)
Centers for Medicare and Medicaid Services—Penelope Meyers, MA, MT(ASCP)SBB
College of American Pathologists—Jean E Forsberg, MD
Food and Drug Administration—Judy E. Ciaraldi, MT(ASCP)SBB, CQA(ASQ);
    Diane Hall, MT(ASCP)SBB; Paul Mintz, MD
ICCBBA—Patricia Distler, MS, MT(ASCP)SBB
Plasma Protein Therapeutics Association—Mary Gustafson, MT(ASCP)SBB
State of California—Ronald N. Harkey

Quality Consultant—Patrick W. Ooley, MS, MT(ASCP), CQA(ASQ)

THE AABB STANDARDS PROGRAM COMMITTEE

Committee Members
Susan D. Roseff, MD, Chair
Julie Allickson, PhD, MS, MT(ASCP)
Jed B. Gorlin, MD, MBA
John H. Holcomb, MD, FACS
Katherine J. Kaherl, MT(ASCP)SBB
Steven Kleinman, MD
Judith Levitt, MT(ASCP)SBB
Mary K. Mount, MT(ASCP)
Kathleen Puca, MD
Mark H. Yazer, MD

Liaisons Representing Other AABB Committees
Accreditation Program Committee–Eva D. Quinley, MT(ASCP)SBB, MS, CQA(ASQ)
Education Program Committee–Virginia M. Vengelen-Tyler, MBA, MT(ASCP)SBB

Representatives from Other Organizations
Armed Services Blood Program Office (DoD)–Col. Richard F. McBride, MT(ASCP)BB
American Society of Hematology–Leslie Silberstein, MD
Canadian Blood Services–Jennifer Biemans, BSc, ART
Food and Drug Administration–Judy E. Ciaraldi, BS, MT(ASCP)SBB, CQA(ASQ);
    Jennifer A. Jones, MBA, CMQ/OE, CQA(ASQ)
Health Canada–Francisca Roseline Agbanyo, PhD
Héma-Québec–Gilles Delage, MD

Quality Consultant
Patrick W. Ooley, MS, MT(ASCP), CQA(ASQ)

PREFACE

The Standards Program Committee (SPC) and the Blood Banks/Transfusion Services Standards Program Unit (BBTS SPU) are pleased to present this 29th edition of *Standards for Blood Banks and Transfusion Services*.

The SPC is the umbrella committee whose primary role is to oversee the creation, development, and revision of all AABB standards to ensure harmonization and consistency in AABB's standard-setting activities. The SPC consists of a committee chair, the chair of the Standards Subcommittee for the Evaluation of International Variances, as well as the chairs of the seven specialty program units.

The BBTS SPU consists of the chair, committee members from the blood banking and transfusion medicine field (including medical and laboratory professionals, and quality experts), liaisons representing other AABB committees, representatives from other organizations, an ethicist, and staff from the AABB national office. The *BBTS Standards* was developed and modified based on input from a variety of sources, including AABB members, the public, and recognized experts in blood banking and transfusion medicine. The BBTS SPU meets during the 2-year revision cycle and has frequent conference calls to discuss requests for variance from each edition of *BBTS Standards* and requests for standards interpretations. Previous editions of the *BBTS Standards* were published on an 18-month cycle, but with this edition going forward, the *BBTS Standards* will now be published on a 24-month cycle, bringing the *BBTS Standards* in line with all other sets of standards for which AABB provides voluntary accreditation.

Although the *BBTS Standards* provides a great amount of technical information concerning the blood banking community, other AABB publications provide specific recommendations. When using this edition of the *BBTS Standards*, having access to the current edition of the AABB *Technical Manual* and the *Circular of Information for the Use of Human Blood and Blood Components* could be of service in understanding and implementing these requirements. Guidance for specific standards that appear in this edition of the *BBTS Standards* will also be published in *Standards Source* through the AABB Community, a forum where AABB members can interact and discuss topics related to their practices in transfusion medicine and cellular therapies. *Standards Source* entries are crafted from member clarification requests and approved variances.

Each edition of the *BBTS Standards* is made possible by the efforts of many talented and dedicated individuals. I wish to express my heartfelt gratitude and appreciation to the 29th edition BBTS SPU committee members, liaisons, representatives, and AABB national office staff for sharing their considerable expertise and time. It has been a privilege and a pleasure to work with everyone! A special thank you is in order for the workgroup chairs Debra Kessler, Kaaron Benson, and Patrick Ooley for their outstanding leadership and diligence. And the process was made easier because of the guidance, skill, and humor of AABB staffers Christopher Bocquet and Eduardo Nunes.

Judith Levitt, MT(ASCP)SBB
Chair, Blood Banks/Transfusion Services Standards Program Unit

INTRODUCTION

The *Standards Blood Banks and Transfusion Services* (*BBTS Standards*) was prepared by the Blood Banks/Transfusion Services Standards Program Unit (BBTS SPU) and the Standards Program Committee (SPC) of the AABB. The goal of the *BBTS Standards* is to maintain and enhance the quality and safety of transfusion and tissue transplantation, and to provide a basis for the AABB Accreditation Program. The following frequently asked questions will help users of this book better understand this 29th edition of *BBTS Standards*:

What activities are covered by the *BBTS Standards*?
For the purposes of this publication, a blood bank stores, collects, processes, and transports human blood intended for transfusion; a transfusion service issues blood and blood components for transfusion. Although these services are typically performed as described, some services may be performed in either a blood bank or a transfusion service. A blood bank or transfusion service may, in addition, store and provide tissue or dispense derivatives. However, it is not the intent of BBTS SPU to require that storage and release of these products be the responsibility of the blood bank or transfusion service. Requirements for these activities are described in this document, and apply only if they are within the scope of the user.

When does this edition go into effect?
The effective date of this edition is April 1, 2014.

Does the *BBTS Standards* contain requirements or recommendations?
The *BBTS Standards* contains requirements to be implemented by AABB-accredited blood banks and transfusion services. A requirement contains the word "shall," which indicates that the statement is mandatory. Failure to meet the requirement would constitute a nonconformance under the AABB Accreditation Program. There are rare instances in which a standard uses the term "may." A statement that uses "may" is not a requirement.

How does this book relate to other laws and regulations?
The *BBTS Standards* was developed on the basis of good medical practice and, when available, scientific and evidence-based data. The requirements in this publication can be followed by a blood bank or transfusion service located anywhere in the world, but they do not preempt your federal, state, and/or local laws and regulations. Accredited facilities must follow the *BBTS Standards* as written to ensure continued AABB accreditation in good standing. Although the majority of the standards here are intended to be

consistent with these applicable laws and requirements, no assurances can be given that compliance with *BBTS Standards* will result in compliance with all applicable laws and requirements. The *BBTS Standards* is not intended as a substitute for legal advice and the content should not be relied upon for legal purposes. Therefore, users must make their own determinations as to how best to ensure compliance with all applicable laws and requirements, including consulting legal counsel familiar with these issues.

Does this publication require me to follow my own local laws and regulations?
Yes. In many standards, the BBTS SPU chose to use the term "specified requirements." This phrase is defined in the glossary to include any applicable requirement under which your service might operate. These could include, but are not limited to, a federal regulation, a customer agreement, a practice standard, the instructions for the intended use of a device, or a requirement of an accrediting organization.

What does the pen symbol (✐) mean?
When the pen symbol precedes a standard, users need to maintain a record of that activity in order to meet the standard. Readers should refer to the reference standard at the end of Chapter 6 to determine what that record must contain.

What other tools are available to help implement the *BBTS Standards?*
Several other resources are available to assist readers. This book also includes:

- A glossary, which reflects the usage of specific words or phrases in the context of the *BBTS Standards*.
- A crosswalk that cross-references the standards in this edition of *BBTS Standards* with those in the previous edition.

  In addition, users of this edition may also want to:

- Visit www.aabb.org for a summary of significant changes to this edition. This summary highlights the most significant changes made to this edition of *BBTS Standards*, and also explains the rationales for any changes. When a public comment is the source of a change, or where the BBTS SPU did not make a change suggested by a comment, an explanation is provided.
- Contact standards@aabb.org for interpretations or to submit a variance request. Variances to standards are effective for the edition of *Standards* for which they are received. Request forms for variances can be found at http://www.aabb.org.

TABLE OF CONTENTS

Table of Contents

1. ORGANIZATION

1.0 Organization

The blood bank or transfusion service shall have a structure that clearly defines and documents the parties responsible for the provision of blood, blood components, tissue, derivatives, and services and the relationship of individuals responsible for key quality functions.

1.1 Executive Management

The blood bank or transfusion service shall have a defined executive management. Executive management shall have:

1) Responsibility and authority for the blood bank's or transfusion service's operations.
2) The authority to establish or make changes to the blood bank's or transfusion service's quality system.
3) The responsibility for compliance with these *BB/TS Standards* and applicable laws and regulations.
4) Participation in management review of the quality system.

1.1.1 Medical Director Qualifications and Responsibilities

The blood bank or transfusion service shall have a medical director who is a licensed physician and qualified by education, training, and/or experience. The medical director shall have responsibility and authority for all medical and technical policies, processes, and procedures—including those that pertain to laboratory personnel and test performance—and for the consultative and support services that relate to the care and safety of donors and/or transfusion recipients. The medical director may delegate these responsibilities to another qualified physician; however, the medical director shall retain ultimate responsibility for medical director duties.

1.2 Quality System

A quality system shall be defined, documented, implemented, and maintained. All personnel shall be trained in its application.

1.2.1 Quality Representative

The quality system shall be under the supervision of a designated person who reports to executive management.

⌀ **1.2.2 Management Reviews**
Management shall assess the effectiveness of the quality system through scheduled management reviews.

1.3 Policies, Processes, and Procedures
Quality and operational policies, processes, and procedures shall be developed and implemented to ensure that the requirements of these *BB/TS Standards* are satisfied. All such policies, processes, and procedures shall be in writing or captured electronically and shall be followed. Standard 5.1.1 applies.

1.3.1 The medical director shall approve all medical and technical policies, processes, and procedures.*

⌀ **1.3.2** Any exceptions to policies, processes, and procedures warranted by clinical situations shall require justification and preapproval by the medical director. Chapter 7, Deviations, Nonconformances, and Adverse Events, applies.

1.4 Emergency Preparedness
The blood bank or transfusion service shall have emergency operation policies, processes, and procedures to respond to the effects of internal and external disasters.

⌀ **1.4.1** The emergency management plan, including emergency communication systems, shall be tested at defined intervals.

1.5 Communication of Concerns
The blood bank or transfusion service shall have a process for personnel to anonymously communicate concerns about quality or safety. Personnel shall be given the option to communicate such concerns either to their facility's executive management, AABB, or both. AABB's contact information shall be readily available to all personnel. Standards 6.1.5 and 9.1 apply.

1.6 Customer Focus
Executive management shall identify the blood bank's or transfusion service's customers and their needs and expectations for products and services.

---

*42 CFR 493.1251(d)

2. RESOURCES

2.0　Resources

The blood bank or transfusion service shall have policies, processes, and procedures to ensure the provision of adequate resources to perform, verify, and manage all activities in the blood bank or transfusion service.

🖉　**2.1　Human Resources**

The blood bank or transfusion service shall have a process to ensure the employment of an adequate number of individuals qualified by education, training, and/or experience. Current job descriptions shall be maintained and shall define appropriate qualifications for each job position.

🖉　**2.1.1　Qualification**

Personnel performing critical tasks shall be qualified to perform assigned activities on the basis of appropriate education, training, and/or experience.

🖉　**2.1.2　Training**

The blood bank or transfusion service shall have a process for identifying training needs and shall provide training for personnel performing critical tasks.

🖉　**2.1.3　Competence**

Evaluations of competence shall be performed before independent performance of assigned activities and at specified intervals.[*]

2.1.3.1　Action shall be taken when competence has not been demonstrated.

🖉　**2.1.4　Personnel Records**

Personnel records for each employee shall be maintained.

🖉　**2.1.4.1**　For those authorized to perform or review critical tasks, records of names, signatures, initials or identification codes, and inclusive dates of employment shall be maintained.

---

[*]42 CFR 493.1235 and 42 CFR 493.1451(b)(8)(9).

3. EQUIPMENT

3.0 Equipment
The blood bank or transfusion service shall identify the equipment that is critical to the provision of blood, blood components, tissue, derivatives, and/or services. The blood bank or transfusion service shall have policies, processes, and procedures to ensure that calibration, maintenance, and monitoring of equipment conforms to these *BBTS Standards* and other specified requirements.

3.1 Selection of Equipment
The blood bank or transfusion service shall have a process to define the selection criteria for equipment.

3.2 Qualification of Equipment
All equipment shall be qualified for its intended use. Equipment repairs and upgrades shall be evaluated and equipment requalified, as appropriate, based on the facility's policies and manufacturer recommendations.

3.2.1 Installation Qualification
Equipment shall be installed per the manufacturer's specifications.

3.2.2 Operational Qualification
The functionality of each piece of equipment and each component of a computer system shall be verified before actual use and shall meet the manufacturer's operational specifications.

3.2.3 Performance Qualification
The blood bank or transfusion service shall demonstrate that equipment performs as expected for its intended use. Performance specifications established by the manufacturer shall be met.

3.3 Use of Equipment
Equipment shall be used in accordance with the manufacturer's written instructions.

3.4 Unique Identification of Equipment
Equipment shall have unique identification. Standard 5.1.6.2 applies.

✐ **3.5 Equipment Monitoring and Maintenance**
The blood bank or transfusion service shall have a process for scheduled monitoring and maintenance of equipment that at a minimum is in accordance with manufacturer's written instructions. The process shall include frequency of checks, check methods, acceptance criteria, and actions to be taken for unsatisfactory results.

3.5.1 Calibration of Equipment
Calibrations and/or adjustments shall be performed using equipment and materials that have adequate accuracy and precision. At a minimum, calibrations and/or adjustments shall be performed as described below unless otherwise indicated by the manufacturer:
1) Before use.
2) After activities that may affect the calibration.
3) At prescribed intervals.

3.5.1.1 There shall be safeguards to prevent equipment from adjustments that would invalidate the calibrated setting. Standard 5.1.3 applies.

3.5.1.2 Calibration procedures shall follow the manufacturer's written instructions and shall include:
1) Instructions for performing calibrations.
2) Acceptance criteria.
3) Actions to be taken when unsatisfactory results are obtained.

3.5.2 Investigation and Follow-up
Investigation and follow-up of equipment malfunctions, failures, or adverse events shall include:
1) Assessment of blood, blood components, tissue, derivatives, and services provided when equipment is found to be out of calibration.
2) Assessment of the effect on donor eligibility and donor and patient safety.
3) Steps to ensure that the equipment is removed from service.
4) Investigation of the malfunction, failure, or adverse event.
5) Steps for requalification of the equipment.
6) Reporting the nature of the malfunction, failure, or adverse event to the manufacturer, when indicated.
Chapter 7, Deviations, Nonconformances, and Adverse Events, applies.

3.6 Storage Devices for Blood, Blood Components, Reagents, Tissue, and Derivatives

3.6.1 Storage devices shall have the capacity and design to ensure that the proper temperature is maintained. Standard 5.1.8.1.3 applies.

3.6.2 Storage temperatures of refrigerators, freezers, and platelet incubators shall be monitored.

3.6.3 If storage devices utilize liquid nitrogen, either liquid nitrogen levels or temperature shall be monitored.

3.7 Alarm Systems

Storage devices for blood, blood components, tissue, and derivatives shall have alarms and shall conform to the following standards (Standard 5.1.3 applies):

3.7.1 The alarm shall be set to activate under conditions that will allow proper action to be taken before blood, blood components, tissue, or derivatives reach unacceptable conditions.

3.7.2 The alarm system in liquid nitrogen freezers shall be activated before the contained liquid nitrogen reaches an unacceptable level.

3.7.3 Activation of the alarm shall initiate a process for immediate investigation and appropriate corrective action.

3.8 Warming Devices for Blood and Blood Components

Warming devices shall be equipped with a temperature-sensing device and a warning system to detect malfunctions and prevent hemolysis or other damage to blood or blood components.

3.9 Information Systems

The blood bank or transfusion service shall have processes to support the implementation and modification of software, hardware, and databases relating to the requirements of these *BBTS Standards*. Standard 5.1.1 applies. These processes shall include:

1) Risk analysis, training, validation, implementation, and evaluation of postimplementation performance.
2) System maintenance and operation.
3) Documentation written in language understandable to the user.

4)   Display and verification of data before final acceptance, when data are added, or when data are amended.

5)   Evaluation, authorization, and documentation of modifications to the system.

3.9.1   Information Systems Records
Records of the following shall be maintained:
1)   Validation of system software, hardware, databases, user-defined tables, electronic data transfer, and/or electronic data receipt.
2)   Fulfillment of applicable life-cycle requirements for internally developed software.[*]
3)   Numerical designation of system versions, if applicable, with inclusive dates of use.
4)   Monitoring of data integrity for critical data elements.

3.9.2   An alternate system shall be maintained to ensure continuous operation in the event that computerized data and computer-assisted functions are unavailable. The alternate system shall be tested periodically. Processes and procedures shall address mitigation of the effects of disasters and include recovery plans.

3.9.3   Personnel responsible for management of information systems shall be responsible for compliance with the regulations that affect their use.

3.9.4   There shall be processes and procedures to support the management of information systems.

3.9.5   A system designed to prevent unauthorized access to computers and electronic records shall be established and followed.

[*]21 CFR 820.30.

FDA Guidance for Industry and FDA Staff: General Principles of Software Validation, January 11, 2002.

FDA Guidance for Industry: Guidance for the Content of Premarket Submissions for Software Contained in Medical Devices, May 11, 2005.

4. SUPPLIER AND CUSTOMER ISSUES

4.0 Supplier and Customer Issues

The blood bank or transfusion service shall have policies, processes, and procedures to evaluate the ability of suppliers of critical materials, equipment, and services to consistently meet specified requirements.

4.1 Supplier Qualification

The blood bank or transfusion service shall evaluate and participate in the selection of suppliers, when possible, before acceptance of an agreement.

4.1.1 When a supplier fails to meet specified requirements, it shall be reported to the management with contracting authority.

4.1.2 Testing or services required by these *BBTS Standards* shall be performed in a laboratory accredited by the AABB or equivalent accrediting body.

4.1.2.1 Laboratory testing shall be performed in a laboratory certified by the Centers for Medicare and Medicaid Services (CMS) and registered with the FDA, if indicated by 21 CFR 610.40(f).

4.2 Agreements

Agreements, or changes to agreements, shall define supplier and customer expectations and shall reflect agreement.

4.2.1 Agreement Review

Agreements and any incorporated changes shall be reviewed and communicated.

4.2.2 The responsibilities for activities covered by these *BB/TS Standards* when more than one facility is involved shall be specified by agreement.

4.3 Incoming Receipt, Inspection, and Testing

Incoming blood, blood components, tissue, derivatives, and critical materials shall be received, inspected, and tested, as necessary, before acceptance or use.

4.3.1 Each container used for collection, preservation, and storage of blood and blood components shall be inspected to ensure that it is intact. The label shall be complete, affixed, and legible.

4.3.2 Critical materials shall meet specified requirements.

4.3.2.1 All containers and solutions used for collection, preservation, and storage and all reagents used for required tests on blood samples shall meet or exceed applicable FDA criteria.[*]

---

[*]See 21 CFR 660, 606.65, 640.2(b), and 640.4(d).

5. PROCESS CONTROL

5.0 Process Control

The blood bank or transfusion service shall have policies and validated processes and procedures that ensure the quality of the blood, blood components, tissue, derivatives, and services. The blood bank or transfusion service shall ensure that these policies, processes, and procedures are carried out under controlled conditions.

5.1 General Elements

5.1.1 Change Control

The blood bank or transfusion service shall have a process to develop new processes or procedures or to change existing ones. This process shall include identification of specifications and verification that specifications have been met. Before implementation, the new or changed processes or procedures shall be validated. Standard 2.1.2 applies.

5.1.2 Proficiency Testing Program

The blood bank or transfusion service shall participate in a proficiency testing program, if available, for testing regulated by the Clinical Laboratory Improvement Amendments and performed by the facility.[*] When a CMS-approved program is not available, there shall be a system for determining the accuracy and reliability of test results. Results shall be reviewed and corrective action taken, where appropriate, when expected results are not achieved.

5.1.3 Quality Control

A program of quality control shall be established that is sufficiently comprehensive to ensure that reagents, equipment, and methods perform as expected. Chapter 9, Process Improvement Through Corrective and Preventive Action, applies.

5.1.3.1 The validity of test results and methods and the acceptability of products or services provided shall be evaluated when quality control failures occur.

---

[*]42 CFR 493.1236.

5.1.3.2   Quality control failures shall be investigated before release of test results, products, or services.

5.1.4   Use of Materials
All materials (including containers and solutions used for collection, processing, preservation, and storage of blood and blood components, and all reagents used for tests) shall be stored and used in accordance with the manufacturer's written instructions and shall meet specified requirements. Standard 3.6 applies.

5.1.4.1   Reagents that are prepared by the facility shall meet or exceed applicable FDA criteria.[*]

5.1.5   Sterility
Aseptic methods shall be employed to minimize the risk of microbial contamination of blood and blood components. Equipment and solutions that come into direct contact with blood or blood components shall be sterile and pyrogen-free. Single-use equipment shall be used whenever possible.

5.1.5.1   The blood bank or transfusion service shall have methods to limit and to detect or inactivate bacteria in all platelet components. Standard 5.6.2 applies.

5.1.5.1.1   Detection methods shall either be cleared or approved by the FDA or be validated to provide sensitivity equivalent to FDA-cleared or -approved methods.

5.1.5.2   When a true-culture positive result is obtained and a sample is available, additional testing to identify the organism shall be performed. Additional testing and follow-up shall be defined. Standards 5.2.4 and 7.1 to 7.1.4 apply.

5.1.6   Identification and Traceability

5.1.6.1   Process or Procedure Steps
For each critical step in collection, processing, compatibility testing and transportation of blood, blood components, tissue, and derivatives, there shall be a mechanism to identify

[*]21 CFR Part 660.

who performed the step and when it was performed. Standard 6.2.4 applies.

5.1.6.2 Traceability
The blood bank or transfusion service shall ensure that all blood, blood components, tissue, derivatives, and critical materials used in their processing, as well as laboratory samples and donor and patient records, are identified and traceable.

5.1.6.3 General Labeling Requirements
The blood bank or transfusion service shall have a labeling process. This process shall include all steps taken to:
1) Identify the original unit, any components, and any component modifications.
2) Complete the required reviews.
3) Attach the appropriate labels. Standard 5.9.1 applies.

5.1.6.3.1 The following requirements shall apply:
1) Labeling of blood and blood component containers shall be in conformance with the most recent version of the United States Industry Consensus Standard for the Uniform Labeling of Blood and Blood Components using ISBT 128.[*] Units conforming to 1985 FDA Uniform Labeling Guidelines are acceptable if collected and labeled before May 1, 2008.[†]
2) The original label and added portions of the label shall be affixed or attached to the container and shall be in clear, eye-readable type. Additionally, the ABO/Rh, donation identification number, product code, and facility identification shall be in machine-readable format.[‡] The label shall include the applicable items required in Reference Standard 5.1.6A,

---

[*]FDA Guidance for Industry: United States Industry Consensus Standard for the Uniform Labeling of Blood and Blood Components Using ISBT 128, version 2.0.0, November 2005, September 22, 2006.
[†]Units collected and labeled before ISBT 128 implementation may be relabeled using Codabar.
[‡]21 CFR 606.121(c)(13).

Requirements for Labeling Blood and Blood Components.

3)   Handwritten additions or changes shall be legible and applied with permanent, moisture-proof ink.

4)   All modifications to component labels shall be specified and controlled.

5)   If a component is modified and new labels are applied, the labeling process shall include a method to ensure the accuracy of all labels, including the donation identification number, ABO/Rh, expiration date (as appropriate), and product name and code.

6)   The labeling process shall include a second check to ensure the accuracy of affixed labels, including the correct donation identification number, ABO/Rh, expiration date (as appropriate), and product name and code.

5.1.6.4   Donor Identification

Blood collection facilities shall confirm donor identity and link the repeat donor to existing donor records.

5.1.6.5   Unit or Tissue Identification

The labeling system shall make it possible to trace any unit of blood, blood component (including those in a pool), or tissue from source to final disposition. The system shall allow recheck of records applying to the specific unit or tissue, including investigation of reported adverse events.

5.1.6.5.1   A unique identification shall be affixed by the collecting or pooling facility to each unit of blood, blood component, and attached container, or a tissue or lot. This identification shall not be obscured, altered, or removed by facilities that subsequently handle the unit.

5.1.6.5.2   If a transfusing facility or other intermediate shipping facility receives a unit labeled with a Codabar Donation Identification Number, then an ISBT 128 Donation Identification or another Codabar Donation

Identification Number may be assigned. The label shall be affixed to the container and shall identify the facility assigning the identification. Any other donation identification number, except that of the original collecting facility, shall be removed, obscured, or obliterated. This requirement does not preclude the use of a patient identification number.

5.1.6.5.3   No more than two donation identifications shall be visible on a blood or product container, one of which shall be that of the original collecting facility. This requirement does not preclude the use of a patient identification number.

5.1.7   Inspection

The blood bank or transfusion service shall have a process to ensure that blood, blood components, tissue, derivatives, and services are inspected at facility-defined stages to verify that specified requirements are met.

5.1.8   Handling, Storage, and Transportation

The blood bank or transfusion service shall have a process to ensure that blood, blood components, tissue, derivatives, samples, and critical materials (including reagents) are handled, stored, and transported in a manner that prevents damage, limits deterioration, and meets requirements contained in Reference Standard 5.1.8A, Requirements for Storage, Transportation, and Expiration.

5.1.8.1   Inventory Management

5.1.8.1.1   The blood bank or transfusion service shall ensure the appropriate segregation of all stored products, including autologous units.

5.1.8.1.2   Tissue and derivatives shall be stored in accordance with the manufacturer's written instructions.

5.1.8.1.3   For storage of blood or blood components, the temperature shall be monitored continuously and recorded at least every 4 hours.

5.1.8.1.3.1 If blood or blood components are stored in an open storage area, the ambient temperature shall be recorded at least every 4 hours.

5.1.8.1.4 Access to storage areas and authorization to remove contents shall be controlled.

5.1.8.2 Transportation
Blood, blood components, tissue,* and derivatives shall be inspected immediately before packing for shipment, and shipped for transfusion or transplantation only if specified requirements are met.

5.1.8.2.1 Containers (eg, portable coolers) used to transport blood and blood components issued for transfusion shall be qualified and the process validated for the appropriate transport temperature and time.

Collection and Production of Components

5.2 Information, Consents, and Notifications

5.2.1 Donor Education
The blood bank shall have procedures to ensure that the following requirements are met for all prospective donors:
1) Donors are given educational materials regarding the donation process.
2) Donors are given educational materials regarding infectious diseases transmitted by blood transfusion.
3) Donors are informed of the importance of providing accurate information.
4) Donors are informed that they should not donate blood in order to obtain infectious disease testing services and that there are circumstances in which testing is not performed.
5) Donors are informed of the importance of withdrawing themselves from the donation process if they believe that their blood is not suitable for transfusion.
6) Donors acknowledge that the educational materials have been read.

---

*21 CFR 1271.3(b), 1271.3(bb), and 21 CFR 1271.15(d).

🖉 **5.2.2** When parental permission is required, the collection facility shall have a process to provide information concerning the donation process to parents or the legally authorized representative of the donor.

🖉 **5.2.3 Donor Consent**
The consent of all donors shall be obtained on the day of donation and before collection. Elements of the donation procedure shall be explained to the prospective donor in understandable terms. The explanation shall include information about risks of the procedure, tests performed to reduce the risks of transmission of infectious diseases to the allogeneic recipient, and requirements to report donor information, including test results, to state or local health departments. The donor shall have an opportunity to ask questions and have them answered and to give or refuse consent for donation. In the case of a minor or a legally incompetent adult, consent shall be addressed in accordance with applicable law.

🖉 **5.2.4 Donor Notification of Abnormal Findings and Test Results**
The medical director shall establish a process to notify all donors (including autologous donors) of any medically significant abnormality detected during the predonation evaluation or as a result of laboratory testing or recipient follow-up. In the case of autologous donors, the referring physician shall also be notified. Appropriate education, counseling, and referral shall be offered.*

5.3 Care of Donors

5.3.1 The collection facility shall have a policy to ensure that the donor qualification process is private and confidential.

5.3.2 The donor shall be observed during the donation and for a length of time thereafter, as defined by the facility's policies and procedures.

5.3.2.1 The collection facility shall have a process for treating donor adverse events and providing for emergency medical care as necessary. Immediate assistance and the necessary equipment and supplies shall be available. Standard 7.3 applies.

---

*21 CFR 630.6.

5.3.3   Postphlebotomy Instructions

5.3.3.1   The collection facility shall provide the donor with written instructions about postphlebotomy care.

5.3.3.2   The collection facility shall provide the donor with written instructions about adverse events that may occur after donation.

5.3.4   Postdonation Information
The collection facility shall provide donors with written instructions on how to notify the collection facility with information relevant to the safety of the donation.

5.3.4.1   The facility shall have a process for managing postdonation information about a donor's eligibility received from the donor or a third party.

5.4   Donor Qualification

5.4.1   Allogeneic Donor Qualification
The prospective donor shall meet the donor qualification requirements contained in Reference Standard 5.4.1A, Requirements for Allogeneic Donor Qualification.

5.4.1.1   Donors implicated in a transfusion-related acute lung injury (TRALI) event or associated with multiple events of TRALI shall be evaluated regarding their continued eligibility to donate.

5.4.1.2   Plasma and whole blood for allogeneic transfusion shall be from males, females who have not been pregnant, or females who have been tested since their most recent pregnancy and results interpreted as negative for HLA antibodies.

5.4.2   Protection of the Recipient
On the day of donation and before collection, the prospective donor's history shall be evaluated and the donor examined to exclude donation by a person with evidence of disease transmissible by blood transfusion or other conditions thought to compromise the suitability of the

blood or blood component. Reference Standard 5.4.1A, Requirements for Allogeneic Donor Qualification, applies.

5.4.2.1 If the collection facility determines that additional clarification or information is needed to evaluate donor eligibility, FDA recommendations* shall apply.

5.4.3 Protection of the Donor

On the day of donation and before collection, the prospective donor's history shall be evaluated and the donor examined to minimize the risk of harm to the donor.

5.4.3.1 The collection facility shall have a program to reduce the risk of reactions in young donors.

5.4.3.2 The collection facility shall ensure that donor red cell losses for all donations and samples collected during any rolling 12-month period do not exceed the loss of red cells permitted for whole blood collections.[†]

5.4.4 Autologous Donor Qualification

Because of the special circumstances related to autologous blood transfusion, rigid criteria for donor selection are not required. In situations where requirements for allogeneic donor selection or collection are not applied, alternate requirements shall be defined and documented by the medical director. Standard 1.3.2 applies. Autologous donor qualification requirements shall include:

5.4.4.1 A medical order from the patient's physician or other authorized health professional to collect blood for autologous use.

---

*FDA Guidance for Industry: Recommendations for Blood Establishments: Training of Back-Up Personnel, Assessment of Blood Donor Suitability and Reporting Certain Changes to an Approved Application, November 2010.

[†]FDA Memorandum to All Registered Blood and Source Plasma Establishments: Donor Deferral Due to Red Blood Cell Loss During Collection of Source Plasma by Automated Plasmapheresis, December 4, 1995.

FDA Guidance for Industry: Technical Correction: Recommendations for Collecting Red Blood Cells by Automated Apheresis Methods, February 13, 2001.

FDA Guidance for Industry and FDA Review Staff: Collection of Platelets by Automated Methods, December 17, 2007.

5.4.4.2   The hemoglobin concentration of the autologous donor's blood shall be ≥11 g/dL, or the hematocrit, if used, shall be ≥33%. Blood obtained by earlobe puncture shall not be used for this determination.

5.4.4.3   All blood collections from the autologous donor shall be completed more than 72 hours before the time of anticipated surgery or transfusion.

5.4.4.4   An autologous donor shall be deferred when he or she has a clinical condition for which there is a risk of bacteremia.

5.4.4.5   The unit shall be reserved for autologous transfusion.

5.5   Additional Apheresis Donor Qualification Requirements

5.5.1   Selection of Donors

With the exception of the donation interval, the standards that apply to allogeneic donor qualification shall apply to the selection of apheresis donors. Donors who do not meet allogeneic donor requirements shall undergo apheresis only when the components are expected to be of particular value to an intended recipient and only when approved by the medical director.

5.5.2   Automated Plasmapheresis Donation

5.5.2.1   Infrequent Plasmapheresis Program

In an "infrequent" plasmapheresis program, donors shall undergo plasmapheresis no more frequently than once every 4 weeks. The plasmapheresis donor shall weigh at least 50 kg (110 lb).[*]

5.5.2.2   Frequent Plasmapheresis Program

In a "frequent" plasmapheresis program, in which plasma is donated more frequently than once every 4 weeks, the FDA requirements for donor testing and evaluation by a physical exam shall be followed.[†]

---

[*]FDA Memorandum to All Registered Blood and Source Plasma Establishments: Revision of FDA Memorandum of August 27, 1982: Requirements for Infrequent Plasmapheresis Donors, March 10, 1995.

[†]21 CFR 640.63 and 21 CFR 640.65 apply.

5.5.2.2.1 Collection shall occur a maximum of two times in a 7-day period and the interval between two collections shall be at least 2 days.[*]

5.5.3 Automated Cytapheresis Donations

5.5.3.1 The interval between procedures for platelet, granulocyte, and leukocyte donors shall be at least 2 days, and the total volume of plasma collected shall not exceed the volume of plasma cleared by the FDA for the instrument. A donor shall undergo the procedure a maximum of two times in a 7-day period, not to exceed 24 times in a rolling 12-month period, except in unusual circumstances as determined by the medical director. Standard 5.4.3.2 applies.[†]

5.5.3.2 If a platelet, granulocyte, or leukocyte donor donates a unit of Whole Blood, at least 8 weeks shall elapse before a subsequent automated cytapheresis procedure, unless the extracorporeal red cell volume of the apheresis machine is less than 100 mL. Standards 5.4.3.2 and 5.5.3.1 apply.

5.5.3.3 If it becomes impossible to return the donor's red cells during apheresis, at least 8 weeks shall elapse before a subsequent apheresis procedure, unless the red cell loss was <200 mL. Standards 5.4.3.2 and 5.5.3.1 apply.[‡]

5.5.3.4 Plateletpheresis Donors
A blood sample shall be collected before each procedure for the determination of the donor's platelet count. If the result is available, it shall be used as the platelet count to qualify the donor.

5.5.3.4.1 If the result of the predonation platelet count is not available, the donor's most recent platelet count may be used to qualify the donor. Triple collections of

---

[*]FDA Memorandum to All Registered Blood Establishments: Volume Limits for Automated Collection of Source Plasma, November 4, 1992.

[†]FDA Guidance for Industry and FDA Review Staff: Collection of Platelets by Automated Methods, December 17, 2007.

[‡]FDA Guidance for Industry: Technical Correction: Recommendations for Collecting Red Blood Cells by Automated Apheresis Methods, February 13, 2001.

Apheresis Platelets may not be collected from first-time donors unless a qualifying platelet count is obtained from a sample collected before donation.

5.5.3.4.2   The results of platelet counts performed before or after a procedure may be used to qualify the donor for the next procedure.

5.5.3.4.3   Plateletpheresis donors with a platelet count of <150,000/µL shall be deferred from plateletpheresis donation until a subsequent platelet count is at least 150,000/µL.*

5.5.3.5   2-Unit Red Blood Cell Apheresis Donors
The donor of a 2-unit Red Blood Cell apheresis collection shall meet specific hemoglobin/hematocrit and weight requirements for the device cleared by the FDA.†

5.5.3.5.1   The donor shall be deferred from all donations for 16 weeks following a 2-unit Red Blood Cell apheresis collection.

5.5.3.5.2   2-Unit Red Blood Cell Collection
The volume of red cells removed from apheresis donors shall not exceed a volume predicted to result in a donor hematocrit of <30% or a hemoglobin <10 g/dL after volume replacement.

5.5.4   Multiple Concurrent Apheresis Collection
The donor eligibility criteria and interval between donations shall meet FDA criteria. The combined volume limits of red cells and plasma removed from the donor shall follow criteria for the FDA-cleared device used.

---

*FDA Guidance for Industry and FDA Review Staff: Collection of Platelets by Automated Methods, December 17, 2007.
†FDA Guidance for Industry: Technical Correction: Recommendations for Collecting Red Blood Cells by Automated Apheresis Methods, February 13, 2001.

5.6 Blood Collection

5.6.1 Methods
Blood shall be collected into a sterile closed system.

5.6.2 Protection Against Contamination
The venipuncture site shall be prepared so as to minimize risk of bacterial contamination. Green soap (USP) shall not be used.

5.6.2.1 Blood collection containers with draw line (inlet) diversion pouches shall be used for any collection of platelets, including whole blood from which platelets are made.

5.6.3 Samples for Laboratory Tests

5.6.3.1 At the time of collection or component preparation, the integral donor tubing shall be filled with anticoagulated blood and sealed in such a manner that it will be available for subsequent compatibility testing.

5.6.3.1.1 The integral donor tubing segments shall be separable from the container without breaking the sterility of the container.

5.6.3.2 Tubes for laboratory tests shall be properly labeled before the donation begins, shall accompany the blood container, and shall be re-identified with the blood container immediately after filling.

5.6.3.3 Storage of samples before testing shall meet the requirements stated in the manufacturer's written instructions for the tests being performed.

5.6.4 Ratio of Blood to Anticoagulant/Preservative Solution
The volume of blood to be collected shall be proportional to the amount of anticoagulant/preservative solution for the collection.

5.6.5 Temperature During Transport
If blood is to be transported from the collection site to the component processing laboratory, it shall be placed in a qualified container having sufficient refrigeration capacity to cool the blood continuously toward a

temperature range of 1 to 10 C until it arrives at the processing laboratory.

5.6.5.1 Whole Blood intended for room temperature component preparation and Apheresis Platelets shall be transported and stored in a manner intended to cool the blood and Apheresis Platelets toward a temperature range of 20 to 24 C.

5.6.6 Additional Apheresis Collection Requirements

5.6.6.1 The process used in performing a phlebotomy and processing the blood shall be designed to ensure safe reinfusion of the autologous nonretained components.

5.6.6.2 Leukapheresis Collection
The collection facility shall have criteria for the administration and dose of any ancillary agents used.

5.6.6.2.1 Drugs to facilitate leukapheresis shall not be used for donors whose medical history suggests that such drugs may exacerbate a medical condition. The collection facility shall have a policy defining the maximal cumulative dose of any sedimenting agent that will be administered to a donor within a given time.

5.6.7 Therapeutic Phlebotomy and Apheresis
Therapeutic phlebotomy and apheresis shall be performed only when ordered by a physician.

5.6.7.1 Units drawn as therapeutic phlebotomies shall not be used for allogeneic transfusion unless one of the following criteria is met:
1) The individual undergoing the therapeutic phlebotomy meets all allogeneic donor criteria and the unit is labeled with the disease/condition of the donor that makes phlebotomy necessary.
2) The indication for therapeutic phlebotomy is hereditary hemochromatosis and the program has received variance approval from the FDA.*

---

*FDA Guidance: Variances for Blood Collection from Individuals with Hereditary Hemochromatosis, August 22, 2001.

5.7 Preparation/Processing of Components

Methods that ensure the quality and safety of components, including aliquots and pooled components, shall be employed.

5.7.1 Seal

If the seal is broken during processing, components shall be considered to have been prepared in an open system and expiration times specified for such components in Reference Standard 5.1.8A, Requirements for Storage, Transportation, and Expiration, apply.

5.7.2 Weld

If a sterile connection device is used to produce sterile welds between two pieces of compatible tubing, the following requirements shall apply:

5.7.2.1 The weld shall be inspected for completeness.

5.7.2.1.1 If the integrity of the weld is complete, the component shall retain original expiration dates or have storage times approved by the FDA.

5.7.2.1.2 If the integrity of the weld is incomplete, the container shall be considered an open system and may be sealed and used with a component expiration as indicated in Reference Standard 5.1.8A, Requirements for Storage, Transportation, and Expiration.

5.7.3 Methods

5.7.3.1 Leukocyte Reduction
Leukocyte-reduced blood and blood components shall be prepared by a method known to reduce the leukocyte number to $<5 \times 10^6$ for Red Blood Cells and Apheresis Platelets[*] and to $<8.3 \times 10^5$ for whole-blood-derived Platelets.[†] Validation and quality control shall demonstrate that at least 95% of units sampled meet this criterion.

---

[*]FDA Guidance for Industry and FDA Review Staff: Collection of Platelets by Automated Methods, December 2007.

[†]FDA Guidance for Industry: Pre-Storage Leukocyte Reduction of Whole Blood and Blood Components Intended for Transfusion, September 2012.

5.7.3.2   Irradiation

Irradiated blood and blood components shall be prepared by a method known to ensure that irradiation has occurred. A method shall be used to indicate that irradiation has occurred with each batch. The intended dose of irradiation shall be a minimum of 25 Gy (2500 cGy) delivered to the central portion of the container. The minimum dose at any point in the components shall be 15 Gy (1500 cGy).* Alternate methods shall be demonstrated to be equivalent.

5.7.3.2.1   Verification of dose delivery shall be performed using a fully loaded canister as follows:
1) Annually for cesium-137 as a radiation source.
2) Semiannually for cobalt-60 as a radiation source.
3) Periodically, as recommended by the manufacturer for alternate sources of radiation.
4) Upon installation, major repairs, or relocation of the irradiator.

5.7.3.3   Pooling

For pooled components, the preparing facility shall maintain records of the ABO/Rh, donation identification number, and collecting facility for each unit in the pool. Standards 5.1.6.5.1 and 5.1.6.5.2 and Reference Standard 5.1.6A, Requirements for Labeling Blood and Blood Components, apply.

5.7.4   Preparation of Specific Components

Reference Standard 5.1.8A, Requirements for Storage, Transportation, and Expiration, applies.

5.7.4.1   RED BLOOD CELLS

Red Blood Cells shall be prepared by separating the red cells from the plasma portion of blood.

5.7.4.1.1   Red Blood Cells without additive solutions shall be prepared using a method known to result in a final hematocrit of ≤80%.

*FDA Guidance: Recommendations Regarding License Amendments and Procedures for Gamma Irradiation of Blood Products, July 22, 1993.

5.7.4.2   FROZEN RED BLOOD CELLS
Frozen Red Blood Cells shall be prepared by a method known to minimize post-thaw hemolysis.

5.7.4.2.1   Red Blood Cells shall be frozen within 6 days of collection, except when rejuvenated. Rare units may be frozen without rejuvenation up to the date of expiration.

5.7.4.3   REJUVENATED RED BLOOD CELLS
Rejuvenated Red Blood Cells shall be prepared by following the manufacturer's written instructions. Rejuvenated Red Blood Cells shall be prepared by a method known to restore 2,3-diphosphoglycerate and adenosine triphosphate to normal levels or above. Reference Standard 5.1.8A, Requirements for Storage, Transportation, and Expiration, applies.

5.7.4.4   DEGLYCEROLIZED RED BLOOD CELLS
Deglycerolized Red Blood Cells shall be prepared by a method known to ensure adequate removal of cryoprotective agents, result in minimal free hemoglobin in the supernatant solution, and yield a mean recovery of $\geq$80% of the preglycerolization red cells following the deglycerolization process.

5.7.4.5   WASHED RED BLOOD CELLS
Washed Red Blood Cells shall be prepared by a method known to ensure that the red cells are washed with a volume of compatible solution that will remove almost all of the plasma.

5.7.4.6   RED BLOOD CELLS LEUKOCYTES REDUCED
Red Blood Cells Leukocytes Reduced shall be prepared by a method known to retain at least 85% of the original red cells and contain $<5 \times 10^6$ residual leukocytes per unit. Standard 5.7.3.1 applies.[*]

---

[*]FDA Guidance for Industry: Pre-Storage Leukocyte Reduction of Whole Blood and Blood Components Intended for Transfusion, September 2012

5.7.4.7 RED BLOOD CELLS LOW VOLUME

When 300 to 404 mL of whole blood is collected into an anticoagulant volume calculated for 450 ± 45 mL or when 333 to 449 mL of whole blood is collected into an anticoagulant volume calculated for 500 ± 50 mL, red cells prepared from the resulting unit shall be labeled Red Blood Cells Low Volume. No other components shall be made from a low-volume collection.

5.7.4.8 APHERESIS RED BLOOD CELLS

Apheresis Red Blood Cells shall be prepared by a method known to ensure a mean collection of ≥60 g of hemoglobin (or 180 mL red cell volume) per unit. At least 95% of the units sampled shall have >50 g of hemoglobin (or 150 mL red cell volume) per unit. Validation and quality control shall demonstrate that these criteria or the criteria specified in the operator's manual are met.

5.7.4.8.1 APHERESIS RED BLOOD CELLS LEUKOCYTES REDUCED

Apheresis Red Blood Cells Leukocytes Reduced shall be prepared by a method known to ensure a final component containing a mean hemoglobin of ≥51 g (or 153 mL red cell volume) and $<5 \times 10^6$ residual leukocytes per unit. At least 95% of units sampled shall have >42.5 g of hemoglobin (or 128 mL red cell volume). Validation and quality control shall demonstrate that these criteria or the criteria specified in the operator's manual are met. Standard 5.7.3.1 applies. Standard 3.3 applies.[*]

5.7.4.9 FRESH FROZEN PLASMA

Fresh Frozen Plasma shall be prepared from a whole blood or apheresis collection and placed at ≤–18 C within the time frame required for the collection, processing, and storage system.

5.7.4.9.1

If a liquid freezing bath is used, the container shall be protected from chemical alteration.

---

[*]FDA Guidance for Industry: Pre-Storage Leukocyte Reduction of Whole Blood and Blood Components Intended for Transfusion, September 2012.

5.7.4.10 **PLASMA FROZEN WITHIN 24 HOURS AFTER PHLEBOTOMY**
Plasma Frozen Within 24 Hours After Phlebotomy shall be prepared from whole blood or apheresis collection. The product prepared from a whole blood collection must be separated and placed at −18 C or below within 24 hours from whole blood collection. When prepared from an apheresis collection the product is stored at 1 to 6 C within 8 hours of collection and frozen at −18 C or colder within 24 hours of collection.

5.7.4.10.1 If a liquid freezing bath is used, the container shall be protected from chemical alteration.

5.7.4.11 **PLASMA FROZEN WITHIN 24 HOURS AFTER PHLEBOTOMY HELD AT ROOM TEMPERATURE UP TO 24 HOURS AFTER PHLEBOTOMY**
Plasma Frozen Within 24 hours After Phlebotomy Held At Room Temperature Up to 24 Hours After Phlebotomy shall be prepared from an apheresis plasma collection. The product can be held at room temperature for up to 24 hours after collection and then frozen at ≤−18 C.

5.7.4.12 **LIQUID PLASMA**
Liquid Plasma shall be prepared by a method known to separate the plasma from the cellular components of the blood.

5.7.4.13 **THAWED PLASMA**
Thawed Plasma shall be prepared from Fresh Frozen Plasma, Plasma Frozen Within 24 Hours After Phlebotomy or Plasma Frozen Within 24 Hours After Phlebotomy Held At Room Temperature Up To 24 Hours After Phlebotomy that has been collected in a closed system.

5.7.4.14 **RECOVERED PLASMA**
Recovered Plasma shall be prepared from donations originally intended for transfusion.

5.7.4.15 **CRYOPRECIPITATED AHF**
Cryoprecipitated AHF shall be prepared by a method known to separate the cold insoluble portion from Fresh Frozen Plasma and result in a minimum of 150 mg of fibrinogen and a minimum of 80 IU of coagulation Factor VIII per container

or unit. In tests performed on prestorage pooled components, the pool shall contain a minimum of 150 mg of fibrinogen and 80 IU of coagulation Factor VIII times the number of components in the pool.

5.7.4.16 PLASMA CRYOPRECIPITATE REDUCED
Plasma Cryoprecipitate Reduced that has been collected in a closed system shall be prepared by refreezing the supernatant plasma that has been used to prepare Cryoprecipitated AHF. It shall be refrozen within 24 hours of thawing the Fresh Frozen Plasma from which it was derived and stored at $\leq$−18 C.

5.7.4.17 THAWED PLASMA CRYOPRECIPITATE REDUCED
Thawed Plasma Cryoprecipitate Reduced shall be prepared from Plasma Cryoprecipitate Reduced.

5.7.4.18 PLATELETS
Validation and quality control of Platelets prepared from Whole Blood shall demonstrate that at least 90% of units sampled contain $\geq 5.5 \times 10^{10}$ platelets and have a pH ≥ 6.2 at the end of allowable storage. FDA criteria apply.[*]

5.7.4.19 PLATELETS LEUKOCYTES REDUCED
Validation and quality control of Platelets Leukocytes Reduced shall demonstrate that at least 75% of units sampled contain $\geq 5.5 \times 10^{10}$ platelets and at least 90% of units sampled have a pH ≥ 6.2 at the end of allowable storage. At a minimum, 95% of units sampled shall contain $<8.3 \times 10^5$ leukocytes. FDA criteria apply.[†]

5.7.4.20 POOLED PLATELETS LEUKOCYTES REDUCED
Pooled Platelets Leukocytes Reduced shall be prepared by a method known to result in a residual leukocyte count $<5 \times 10^6$. Standard 5.7.4.19 applies.

---

[*]21 CFR 640.25(b).
[†]21 CFR 640.25(b).
FDA Guidance for Industry: Pre-Storage Leukocyte Reduction of Whole Blood and Blood Components Intended for Transfusion, September 2012.

5.7.4.21 APHERESIS PLATELETS
Validation and quality control of Apheresis Platelets shall demonstrate that at least 90% of units sampled contain $\geq 3.0 \times 10^{11}$ platelets and, at the end of allowable storage or at the time of issue, have a pH ≥ 6.2. FDA criteria apply.[*†]

5.7.4.22 APHERESIS PLATELETS LEUKOCYTES REDUCED
Validation and quality control shall demonstrate that 90% of units sampled contain $\geq 3.0 \times 10^{11}$ platelets and, at the end of allowable storage or at the time of issue, have a pH ≥ 6.2. FDA criteria apply.[‡] At a minimum, 95% of units sampled shall contain a residual leukocyte count $<5 \times 10^6$.[§]

5.7.4.23 APHERESIS PLATELETS PLATELET ADDITIVE SOLUTION ADDED LEUKOCYTES REDUCED
Apheresis Platelets Platelet Additive Solution Added Leukocytes Reduced shall be collected by apheresis and suspended in variable amounts of plasma and an approved platelet additive solution. Validation and quality control shall demonstrate that at least 90% of units sampled contain $\geq 3.0 \times 10^{11}$ platelets. At a minimum, 95% of units sampled shall contain a residual leukocyte count $<5 \times 10^6$.

5.7.4.24 APHERESIS GRANULOCYTES
Unless prepared for neonates, Apheresis Granulocytes shall be prepared by a method known to yield a minimum of 1.0×10^{10} granulocytes in at least 75% of the units tested. Product requirements for neonates shall be defined by the medical director.

[*]21 CFR 640.25(b).
[†]FDA Guidance for Industry and FDA Review Staff: Collection of Platelets by Automated Methods, December 17, 2007.
[‡]21 CFR 640.25(b).
[§]FDA Guidance for Industry and FDA Review Staff: Collection of Platelets by Automated Methods, December 17, 2007.

5.8 Testing of Donor Blood

5.8.1 Determination of ABO Group for All Collections
The ABO group shall be determined for each collection by testing the red cells with anti-A and anti-B reagents and by testing the serum or plasma for expected antibodies with A_1 and B reagent red cells.

5.8.2 Determination of Rh Type for All Collections
The Rh type shall be determined for each collection with anti-D reagent. If the initial test with anti-D is negative, the blood shall be tested using a method designed to detect weak D. When either test is positive, the label shall read "Rh POSITIVE." When the tests for both D and weak D are negative, the label shall read "Rh NEGATIVE."

5.8.3 Detection of Unexpected Antibodies to Red Cell Antigens for Allogeneic Donors

5.8.3.1 Serum or plasma from donors shall be tested for unexpected antibodies to red cell antigens.

5.8.3.2 Methods for testing shall be those that demonstrate clinically significant red cell antibodies.[*]

5.8.3.3 A control system appropriate to the method of testing shall be used. Standard 5.1.3 applies.

5.8.4 Red Cell Antigens Other than ABO and RhD
Units may be labeled as antigen negative, without testing the current donation, if units from two previous separate donations were tested by the collection facility and found to be concordant.

5.8.5 Tests Intended to Prevent Disease Transmission by Allogeneic Donations
A sample of blood from each allogeneic donation shall be tested for HBV DNA, HBsAg, anti-HBc, anti-HCV, HCV RNA, anti-HIV-1/2, HIV-1 RNA, anti-HTLV-I/II, WNV RNA, and syphilis by a serologic test. Each donor shall be tested at least once for antibodies to *Trypanosoma cruzi*. Blood and blood components shall not be distributed or issued for transfusion unless the results of these tests are negative, except in the case of a test for syphilis that has been shown to have a biological

[*]21 CFR 606.151(d).

false-positive result. Units with biological false-positive results shall be labeled in accordance with FDA requirements.* Standard 5.2.4 applies.

5.8.5.1 If, due to urgent need, blood or blood components are distributed or issued before completion of these tests, a notation that testing is not completed shall appear conspicuously on an attached label or tie tag. Required tests shall be completed and results reported to the transfusion service as soon as possible.

5.8.5.2 For a cytapheresis donor dedicated to the support of a specific patient, testing required by Standard 5.8.5 shall be performed at the first donation and at least every 30 days thereafter.†

5.8.6 Tests Intended to Prevent Disease Transmission by Autologous Donations
Autologous blood or components that will be transfused outside the collection facility shall be tested for HBV DNA, HBsAg, anti-HBc, anti-HCV, HCV RNA, anti-HIV-1/2, HIV-1 RNA, anti-HTLV-I/II, WNV RNA, and syphilis by a serologic test. Each donor shall be tested at least once for antibodies to *T. cruzi*. These tests shall be performed before shipping on at least the first unit collected during each 30-day period.‡

5.8.6.1 The patient's physician and the donor-patient shall be informed of any medically significant abnormalities discovered. Standard 5.2.4 applies.§

5.8.7 Quarantine and Disposition of Units from Prior Collections
The blood bank or transfusion service shall have a process that is in accordance with FDA requirements and recommendations for quarantine and disposition of prior collections when a repeat donor has a reactive screening test for HBV DNA, HBsAg, anti-HBc, anti-HCV, HCV

---

*FDA Memorandum to All Registered Blood Establishments: Clarification of FDA Recommendations for Donor Deferral and Product Distribution Based on the Result of Syphilis Testing, December 12, 1991.
21 CFR 610.40.
†21 CFR 610.40(c)(1).
‡21 CFR 610.40(d).
§21 CFR 630.6(d).

RNA, anti-HIV-1/2, HIV-1 RNA, anti-HTLV-I/II, WNV RNA, or *T. cruzi* antibodies.[*]

5.9 Final Labeling

The blood bank or transfusion service shall have a process to ensure that all specified requirements have been met at final labeling.

5.9.1 Testing and acceptability criteria shall be defined, and there shall be evidence that all records relating to testing and acceptability criteria for the current donation, and the facility's deferral registry, have been reviewed.

5.9.2 The component shall be physically inspected for container integrity and normality of appearance.

5.9.3 ABO/Rh typing shall be compared to a historical type, if available. Discrepancies shall be resolved before release.

---

[*]21 CFR 610.46, 610.47, and 610.48.

FDA Memorandum to All Registered Blood Establishments: Revised Recommendations for the Prevention of Human Immunodeficiency Virus (HIV) Transmission by Blood and Blood Products, April 23, 1992.

FDA Memorandum to All Registered Blood and Plasma Establishments: Recommendations for the Quarantine and Disposition of Units from Prior Collection from Donors with Repeatedly Reactive Screening Tests for Hepatitis B Virus (HBV), Hepatitis C Virus (HCV) and Human T Lymphotropic Virus Type I (HTLV-I), July 19, 1996.

FDA Guidance for Industry: Donor Screening for Antibodies to HTLV II, August 15, 1997.

FDA Guidance for Industry: Use of Nucleic Acid Tests to Reduce the Risk of Transmission of West Nile Virus from Donors of Whole Blood and Blood Components Intended for Transfusion, November 6, 2009.

FDA Guidance for Industry: Nucleic Acid Testing (NAT) for Human Immunodeficiency Virus Type 1 (HIV-1) and Hepatitis C Virus (HCV): Testing, Product Disposition, and Donor Deferral and Reentry, May 2010.

FDA Guidance for Industry: Use of Serological Tests to Reduce the Risk of Transmission of Trypanosoma cruzi Infection in Whole Blood and Blood Components Intended for Transfusion, December 2010.

FDA Guidance for Industry: Lookback' for Hepatitis C Virus (HCV): Product Quarantine, Consignee Notification, Further Testing, Product Disposition, and Notification of Transfusion Recipients Based on Donor Test Results Indicating Infection with HCV, December 2010.

FDA Guidance for Industry: Use of Nucleic Acid Tests on Pooled and Individual Samples from Donors of Whole Blood and Blood Components, Including Source Plasma, to Reduce the Risk of Transmission of Hepatitis B Virus, October 2012.

🖉 **5.9.4**   The facility shall ensure that blood and blood components from ineligible donors are quarantined and are not issued for transfusion.

5.9.5   There shall be a method to confirm that the ABO/Rh label is correct. Confirmation shall be performed after the ABO and Rh label has been affixed to the units.

  5.9.5.1   When an information system is used, it shall be validated to prevent the release of ABO- and Rh-mislabeled components.

  5.9.5.2   The confirmation process shall be completed before release.

5.10 Final Inspection
The blood bank or transfusion service shall have a process to ensure that blood, blood components, tissue, derivatives, or services meet specified requirements, including appearance before distribution or issue.

Transfusion-Service-Related Activities

5.11 Samples and Requests
Identifying information for the patient and the sample shall correspond and be confirmed at the time of collection using two independent identifiers.

🖉 **5.11.1 Requests**
Requests for blood, blood components, tests, tissue, and derivatives and records accompanying samples from the patient shall contain sufficient information to uniquely identify the patient, including two independent identifiers. The transfusion service shall accept only complete, accurate, and legible requests.

🖉   **5.11.1.1**   A physician or other authorized health professional shall order blood, blood components, tests, tissue, and derivatives.

5.11.2 Patient Samples
Patient samples shall be identified with an affixed label bearing sufficient information for unique identification of the patient, including two independent identifiers.

5.11.2.1 The completed label shall be affixed to the sample container before the person who obtained the sample leaves the side of the patient.

5.11.2.2 There shall be a mechanism to identify the date of sample collection and the individual(s) who collected the sample from the patient.

5.11.2.3 The transfusion service shall accept only those samples that are completely, accurately, and legibly labeled.

5.11.3 Identifying Information
The transfusion service shall confirm that all identifying information on the request is in agreement with that on the sample label. In case of discrepancy or doubt, another sample shall be obtained.

5.11.4 Retention of Blood Samples
Patient samples and a segment from any red-cell-containing component(s) shall be stored at refrigerated temperatures for at least 7 days after transfusion.

5.12 Serologic Confirmation of Donor Blood ABO/Rh (including autologous units)
Before transfusion, the ABO group of each unit of Whole Blood, Red Blood Cell, and Granulocyte component and the Rh type of such units labeled as Rh negative shall be confirmed by a serologic test from an integrally attached segment. Confirmatory testing for weak D is not required.

5.12.1 Discrepancies shall be reported to the collecting facility and shall be resolved before issue of the blood for transfusion. Standards 7.1.1 and 7.1.2 apply.

5.13 Serologic Confirmation of Donor Blood Red Cell Antigens Other Than ABO/Rh
Red Blood Cell products labeled as negative for red cell antigens other than ABO and RhD do not require repeat testing for the labeled antigens.

5.14 Pretransfusion Testing of Patient Blood
Pretransfusion tests for allogeneic transfusion shall include ABO group and Rh type. In addition, for Whole Blood, Red Blood Cell, and Granulocyte components, pretransfusion testing for unexpected antibodies to red cell antigens shall be performed.

5.14.1 ABO Group

The ABO group shall be determined by testing the red cells with anti-A and anti-B reagents and by testing the serum or plasma for expected antibodies with A_1 and B reagent red cells. If a discrepancy is detected and transfusion is necessary before resolution, only group O Red Blood Cells shall be issued.

5.14.2 Rh Type

Rh type shall be determined with anti-D reagent. The test for weak D is unnecessary when testing the patient.

5.14.3 Unexpected Antibodies to Red Cell Antigens

Methods of testing shall be those that demonstrate clinically significant antibodies. They shall include incubation at 37 C preceding an anti-globulin test using reagent red cells that are not pooled.

5.14.3.1 When clinically significant antibodies are detected, additional testing shall be performed.

5.14.3.2 If the patient has been transfused in the preceding 3 months with blood or a blood component containing allogeneic red cells, if the patient has been pregnant within the preceding 3 months, or if the history is uncertain or unavailable, a sample shall be obtained from the patient within 3 days of the scheduled transfusion. Day 0 is the day of draw.

5.14.3.3 In patients with previously identified clinically significant antibodies, methods of testing shall be those that identify additional clinically significant antibodies.

5.14.3.4 A control system appropriate to the method of testing shall be used. Standard 5.1.3 applies.

5.14.4 Pretransfusion Testing for Autologous Transfusion

Pretransfusion testing for autologous transfusion shall include ABO group and Rh type on the patient sample. Standard 5.11 applies.

5.14.5 Comparison with Previous Records

There shall be a process to ensure that the historical records for the following have been reviewed:
1) ABO group and Rh type.

2)   Difficulty in blood typing.
3)   Clinically significant antibodies.
4)   Significant adverse events to transfusion.
5)   Special transfusion requirements.

These records shall be compared to current results, and any discrepancies shall be investigated and appropriate action taken before a unit is issued for transfusion.

5.15 Selection of Compatible Blood and Blood Components for Transfusion

5.15.1   Recipients shall receive ABO group-specific Whole Blood or ABO group-compatible Red Blood Cell components.

5.15.2   Rh-negative recipients shall receive Rh-negative Whole Blood or Red Blood Cell components.

5.15.2.1   The transfusion service shall have a policy for the use of Rh-positive red-cell-containing components in Rh-negative recipients. Standard 5.30 applies.

5.15.3   When clinically significant red cell antibodies are detected or the recipient has a history of such antibodies, Whole Blood or Red Blood Cell components shall be prepared for transfusion that do not contain the corresponding antigen and are serologically crossmatch-compatible.

5.15.4   The transfusion service shall have a policy concerning transfusion of components containing significant amounts of incompatible ABO antibodies or unexpected red cell antibodies.

5.15.5   The red cells in Apheresis Granulocytes and Platelets shall be ABO-compatible with the recipient's plasma and be crossmatched as in Standard 5.16 unless the component is prepared by a method known to result in a component containing <2 mL of red cells. The donor blood cells for the crossmatch may be obtained from a sample collected at the time of donation.

5.16 Crossmatch

5.16.1   Serologic Crossmatch
Before issue, a sample of the recipient's serum or plasma shall be crossmatched against a sample of donor cells from an integrally attached Whole Blood or Red Blood Cell segment. The crossmatch

shall use methods that demonstrate ABO incompatibility and clinically significant antibodies to red cell antigens and shall include an antiglobulin test as described in Standard 5.14.3.

5.16.1.1   If no clinically significant antibodies were detected in tests performed in Standard 5.14.3 and there is no record of previous detection of such antibodies, at a minimum, detection of ABO incompatibility shall be performed.

5.16.2   Use of Computer to Detect ABO Incompatibility
If a computer system is used as a method to detect ABO incompatibility, the following requirements shall be met:

5.16.2.1   The computer system has been validated on site to ensure that only ABO-compatible Whole Blood or Red Blood Cell components have been selected for transfusion.

5.16.2.2   Two determinations of the recipient's ABO group as specified in Standard 5.14.1 are made—one on a current sample, and the second by one of the following methods:
1) Testing a second current sample.
2) Comparison with previous records.
3) Retesting the same sample.
Standard 5.11 applies.

5.16.2.3   The system contains the donation identification number, component name, ABO group, and Rh type of the component; the confirmed unit ABO group; the two unique recipient identifiers; recipient ABO group, Rh type, and antibody screen results; and interpretation of compatibility.

5.16.2.4   A method exists to verify correct entry of data before release of blood or blood components.

5.16.2.5   The system contains logic to alert the user to discrepancies between the donor ABO group and Rh type on the unit label and those determined by blood group confirmatory tests and to ABO incompatibility between the recipient and the donor unit.[*]

---

[*]FDA Guidance for Industry: Computer Crossmatch (Computer Analysis of the Compatibility between the Donor's Cell Type and the Recipient's Serum or Plasma Type), April 2011.

5.17 Special Considerations for Neonates

🖉 **5.17.1** An initial pretransfusion sample shall be tested to determine ABO group and Rh type. For ABO, only anti-A and anti-B reagents are required. The Rh type shall be determined as in Standard 5.14.2. The serum or plasma of either the neonate or the mother may be used to perform the test for unexpected antibodies as in Standard 5.14.3.

5.17.1.1 Repeat ABO grouping and Rh typing may be omitted for the remainder of the neonate's hospital admission or until the neonate reaches the age of 4 months, whichever is sooner.

5.17.1.2 If the initial screen for red cell antibodies is negative, it is unnecessary to crossmatch donor red cells for the initial or subsequent transfusions. Repeat testing may be omitted for the remainder of the neonate's hospital admission or until the neonate reaches the age of 4 months, whichever is sooner. Standard 5.17.2 applies.

🖉 **5.17.1.3** If the initial antibody screen demonstrates clinically significant unexpected red cell antibodies, units shall be prepared for transfusion that either do not contain the corresponding antigen or are compatible by antiglobulin crossmatch until the antibody is no longer demonstrable in the neonate's serum or plasma.

🖉 **5.17.2** If a non-group-O neonate is to receive non-group-O Red Blood Cells that are not compatible with the maternal ABO group, the neonate's serum or plasma shall be tested for anti-A or anti-B.

5.17.2.1 Test methods shall include an antiglobulin phase using either donor or reagent A_1 or B red cells. Standard 5.14.3.4 applies.

5.17.2.2 If anti-A or anti-B is detected, Red Blood Cells lacking the corresponding ABO antigen shall be transfused.

🖉 ### 5.18 Special Considerations for Intrauterine Transfusion
The blood bank or transfusion service shall have a policy regarding intrauterine transfusion including a mechanism to ensure that fetal transfusion and fetal blood type, when performed, is differentiated from that of the mother.

5.19 Selection of Compatible Blood and Blood Components in Special Circumstances

Once it has been determined that a patient has special transfusion requirements, there shall be a mechanism to ensure that all future blood or blood components for that patient meet the special transfusion requirements for as long as clinically indicated.

5.19.1 Leukocyte-Reduced Components

The blood bank or transfusion service shall have a policy regarding transfusion of leukocyte-reduced components.

5.19.2 Cytomegalovirus

The blood bank or transfusion service shall have a policy regarding transfusion of cellular components selected or processed to reduce the risk of cytomegalovirus (CMV) transmission.

5.19.3 Irradiation

The blood bank or transfusion service shall have a policy regarding the transfusion of irradiated components.

5.19.3.1 At a minimum, cellular components shall be irradiated when:

5.19.3.1.1 A patient is identified as being at risk for transfusion-associated graft-vs-host disease.

5.19.3.1.2 The donor of the component is a blood relative of the recipient.

5.19.3.1.3 The donor is selected for HLA compatibility, by typing or crossmatching.

5.19.4 Hemoglobin S

The blood bank or transfusion service shall have a policy regarding indications for the transfusion of Red Blood Cells or Whole Blood known to lack hemoglobin S.

5.19.5 Massive Transfusion

The blood bank or transfusion service shall have a policy regarding compatibility testing when, within 24 hours, a patient has received an amount of blood approximating or greater than the total blood volume.

5.19.6 Specially Selected Platelets
The blood bank or transfusion service shall have a policy regarding indications for specially selected platelet requirements—for example, HLA-matched, crossmatch-compatible, HLA antigen-negative, and HPA antigen-negative platelets.

5.20 Preparation of Tissue
The facility shall have policies, processes, and procedures to ensure that any preparation steps performed before dispensing tissue are in accordance with the source facility's processes and procedures. The following information shall be maintained:
1) Type of tissue.
2) Numeric or alphanumeric identifier.
3) Quantity.
4) Expiration date and, if applicable, time.
5) Identity of personnel who prepared the tissue and the date of preparation.

5.21 Preparation of Derivatives
The facility shall have policies, processes, and procedures to ensure that any preparation steps performed before dispensing derivatives are in accordance with the source facility's processes and procedures. The following information shall be maintained:
1) Type of derivative.
2) Lot number.
3) Quantity.
4) Expiration date and, if applicable, time.
5) Identity of personnel who prepared the derivative and the date of preparation.

5.22 Final Inspection Before Issue
Blood, blood components, tissue, and derivatives shall be inspected at the time of issue.

5.22.1 Transfusion Recipient Blood Container Identification
A blood container shall have an attached label or tie tag indicating:
1) The intended recipient's two independent identifiers.
2) Donation identification number or pool number.
3) Interpretation of compatibility tests, if performed.

5.23 Issue of Blood and Blood Components

At the time a unit is issued, there shall be a final check of transfusion service records and each unit of blood or blood component. Verification shall include:

1) The intended recipient's two independent identifiers, ABO group, and Rh type.
2) The donation identification number, the donor ABO group, and, if required, the Rh type.
3) The interpretation of crossmatch tests, if performed.
4) Special transfusion requirements, if applicable.
5) The expiration date and, if applicable, time.
6) The date and time of issue.

5.24 Issue of Tissue and Derivatives

The following information shall be verified:

1) The manufacturer's package insert documents are issued with the product or listed on the product contents list.
2) The product quantity and name are consistent with the request.
3) The record of final inspection of the product.
4) If tissue or derivatives are issued for a specific patient, the intended recipient's two independent identifiers.
5) The expiration date and, if applicable, time.
6) The date and time of issue.

5.25 Discrepancy Resolution

The blood bank or transfusion service shall have a process to confirm agreement of the identifying information, the records, the blood or blood component, and the request. Discrepancies shall be resolved before issue.

5.26 Reissue of Blood, Blood Components, Tissue, and Derivatives

Blood, blood components, tissue, or derivatives that have been returned to the blood bank or transfusion service shall be accepted into inventory for reissue only if the following conditions have been met:

1) The container closure has not been disturbed.
2) The appropriate temperature has been maintained.
3) For Red Blood Cell components, at least one sealed segment of integral donor tubing has remained attached to the container. Removed segments shall be reattached only after confirming that the tubing identification numbers on both the removed segment(s) and the container are identical.
4) The records indicate that the blood, blood component, tissue, or derivatives have been inspected and that they are acceptable for reissue.

5.27 Urgent Requirement for Blood and Blood Components

The blood bank or transfusion service shall have a process for the provision of blood and blood components before completion of tests listed in Standards 5.8.4, 5.14, 5.14.1, 5.14.2, 5.14.3, and 5.16 when a delay in transfusion could be detrimental to the patient. Standards 5.8.5.1, 5.12, and 7.0 to 7.2 apply.

5.27.1 Recipients whose ABO group is not known shall receive group O Red Blood Cells. Standard 5.14.1 applies.

5.27.2 If blood is issued before completion of compatibility testing, recipients whose ABO group has been determined as in Standard 5.14.1 by the transfusing facility shall receive only ABO group-specific Whole Blood or ABO group-compatible Red Blood Cell components.

5.27.3 The container tie tag or label shall indicate in a conspicuous fashion that compatibility and/or infectious disease testing was not completed at the time of issue.

5.27.4 Compatibility testing shall be completed expeditiously using a patient sample collected as early as possible in the transfusion sequence. Standard 5.19.5 applies.

5.27.5 The records shall contain a signed statement from the requesting physician indicating that the clinical situation was sufficiently urgent to require release of blood before completion of compatibility testing or infectious disease testing.

5.27.5.1 The transfusion service medical director and the recipient's physician shall be notified immediately of abnormal test results that may affect patient safety.

5.28 Administration of Blood and Blood Components

There shall be a protocol for the administration of blood and blood components, including the use of infusion devices and ancillary equipment, and the identification, evaluation, and reporting of adverse events related to transfusion. The medical director shall participate in the development of these protocols. The protocol shall be consistent with the Circular of Information for the Use of Human Blood and Blood Components. Standard 7.4 applies.

🖉 **5.28.1 Recipient Consent**
The blood bank or transfusion service medical director shall participate in the development of policies, processes, and procedures regarding recipient consent for transfusion.

5.28.1.1 At a minimum, elements of consent shall include all of the following:
1) A description of the risks, benefits, and treatment alternatives (including nontreatment).
2) The opportunity to ask questions.
3) The right to accept or refuse transfusion.

5.28.2 Transfusions shall be prescribed and administered under medical direction.

🖉 **5.28.3** After issue and immediately before transfusion, the following information shall be verified:
1) The intended recipient's two independent identifiers, ABO group, and Rh type.
2) The donation identification number, the donor ABO group, and, if required, the Rh type.
3) The interpretation of crossmatch tests, if performed.
4) Special transfusion requirements are met, if applicable.
5) The unit has not expired.

🖉 **5.28.4** The transfusionist and one other individual (or an electronic identification system) shall, in the presence of the recipient positively identify the recipient and match the blood component to the recipient through the use of two independent identifiers.

5.28.5 All identification attached to the container shall remain attached until the transfusion has been terminated.

5.28.6 The patient shall be observed for potential adverse events during the transfusion and for an appropriate time thereafter. Standard 7.4 applies.

5.28.7 Specific written instructions concerning possible adverse events shall be provided to the patient or a responsible caregiver when direct medical observation or monitoring of the patient will not be available after transfusion.

5.28.8 Blood and blood components shall be transfused through a sterile, pyrogen-free transfusion set that has a filter designed to retain particles potentially harmful to the recipient.

5.28.9 Addition of Drugs and Solutions
With the exception of 0.9% sodium chloride (USP), drugs or medications shall not be added to blood or blood components unless one of the following conditions is met:
1) They have been approved for this use by the FDA.
2) There is documentation available to show that the addition is safe and does not adversely affect the blood or blood component.

5.28.10 Granulocytes
Leukocyte reduction filters or microaggregate filters shall not be used. Standard 5.28.8 applies.

5.29 Medical Record Documentation

5.29.1 The patient's medical record shall include the transfusion order, documentation of patient consent, the name of the component, the donation identification number, the date and time of transfusion, pre- and posttransfusion vital signs, the amount transfused, the identification of the transfusionist, and, if applicable, transfusion-related adverse events.

5.29.2 For recipients of tissue, the recipient's medical record shall include the type of tissue, the numeric or alphanumeric identifier, the quantity, the expiration date and the date of use, personnel using the tissue, and, if applicable, related adverse events.

5.29.3 For recipients of derivatives, the recipient's medical record shall include the product name, the lot number, the quantity, and the date and time of administration, individuals administering the derivative, and, if applicable, related adverse events.

5.30 Rh Immune Globulin
The transfusion service shall have a policy for Rh Immune Globulin prophylaxis for Rh-negative patients who have been exposed to Rh-positive red cells.

5.30.1 Interpretation criteria shall be established to prevent the mistyping of an Rh-negative patient as Rh positive due to exposure to Rh-positive red cells.

5.30.2 Women who are pregnant or who have been pregnant recently shall be considered for Rh Immune Globulin administration when all of the following apply:
1) The woman's test for D antigen is negative. A test for weak D is not required.
2) The woman is not known to be actively immunized to the D antigen.
3) The Rh type of the fetus/infant is unknown or the type of the fetus/infant is positive when tested for D or weak D. Weak D testing is required when the test for D is negative.

5.30.3 There shall be a process to ensure that an adequate dose of Rh Immune Globulin is administered.

5.30.4 Rh Immune Globulin shall be administered as soon as possible after exposure.

5.30.5 Patients who have received Rh Immune Globulin shall be evaluated to determine the need for additional treatment.

Reference Standard 5.1.6A—Requirements for Labeling Blood and Blood Components

Item No.	Labeling Item	Collection or Preparation	Final Component	Pooled
1	Name of blood component or intended component[1]	NR	R	R
2	Donation identification number[1]	R	R	R
3	Identity of anticoagulant[2] or other preservative solution	R	R	R
4	Identity of sedimenting agent, if applicable	NR	R	NA
5	Approximate volume[3]	NR	R	R, total
6	Facility collecting component[1]	NR	R	NR
7	Facility modifying component[4]	NA	R, if leaves the facility	R[1]
8	Storage temperature	NA	R	R
9	Expiration date and, when appropriate, time	NA	R	R
10	ABO group and Rh type[1,5]	NA	R	See line 18
11	Specificity of unexpected red cell antibodies[6,7]	NA	R[2]	R
12	Instructions to the transfusionist:[8]	NR	R	R

1. See *Circular of Information for the Use of Human Blood and Blood Components*
2. "Properly identify intended recipient"
3. "This product may transmit infectious agents"
4. "Rx Only"

(Continued)

Reference Standard 5.1.6A—Requirements for Labeling Blood and Blood Components (Continued)

Item No.	Labeling Item	Collection or Preparation	Final Component	Pooled
13	Phrase: "Volunteer Donor," if applicable	NR	R	R
14	Phrase: "Paid Donor," if applicable	R	R	R
15	CMV seronegative, if applicable	NR	R	R
16	Indication that the unit is low volume, if applicable.	NR	R	NA
17	Number of units in pool[6]	NA	NA	R
18	ABO and Rh of units in pool[5,9]	NA	NA	R
19	Red cell antigens other than ABO or RhD, if applicable[6]	NA	R	NA
	Additional Autologous Labeling Requirements			
20	Phrase: "For autologous use only"[6]	R	R	R
21	Recipient name, identification number, and, if available, name of facility where patient is to be transfused[6]	R	R	R
22	Biohazard label, if applicable[10]	NR	R	R
23	Phrase: "Donor untested," if applicable[11]	NR	R	NA
24	Phrase: "Donor tested within the last 30 days," if applicable[12]	NR	R	NA
	Additional Dedicated Donor Labeling Requirements			
25	Intended recipient information label	R	R	NA

26	Donor tested within the last 30 days, if applicable[12]	NR	R	NA
27	Biohazard label, if applicable[10]	NR	R	R

Labeling Requirements for Recovered Plasma[11]

28	"Caution: For Manufacturing Use Only"	NA	R	R
29	Biohazard label, if applicable	NR	R	R
30	"Not for Use in Products Subject to License Under Section 351 of the Public Health Service Act" (Applicable to plasma not meeting requirements for manufacture into licensable products)	NA	R	R
31	In lieu of expiration date, the date of collection of the oldest material in the container	R	R	R

R = required; NR = not required; NA = not applicable.
[1]Must be machine-readable (see Standard 5.1.6.3.1).
[2]Not required for cryoprecipitate, frozen, deglycerolized, rejuvenated, or washed Red Blood Cells.
[3]For platelets, low-volume Red Blood Cells, plasma, pooled components, and components prepared by apheresis, the approximate volume in the container.
[4]Includes irradiation, if applicable.
[5]Rh type not required for cryoprecipitate or pooled cryoprecipitate.
[6]The facility has the option of putting information on a tie tag or label.
[7]Specificity of antibodies is not required for autologous units.
[8]Wording may be different outside of the United States.
[9]For pooled cryoprecipitate, plasma, or platelets of mixed types, a pooled type label is acceptable. The specific ABO group and Rh types of units in the pool may be put on a tie tag. Standard 5.7.3.3 applies.

(Continued)

Reference Standard 5.1.6A—Requirements for Labeling Blood and Blood Components (Continued)

[10]Biohazard labels for autologous units or allogeneic units from a dedicated donor shall be used for the following test results:

Test	Test Result
HBsAg	Repeatedly reactive
Anti-HBc	Repeatedly reactive
HBV NAT	Positive or reactive
Anti-HCV	Repeatedly reactive
HCV NAT	Positive or reactive
Anti-HIV-1/2	Repeatedly reactive
HIV-1 NAT	Positive or reactive
Anti-HTLV-I/II	Repeatedly reactive
WNV NAT	Positive or reactive
Syphilis	Reactive screening test with a positive confirmatory test or no confirmatory test

When performed:
T. cruzi Antibody Screening   Repeatedly reactive

[11]Donor not tested for evidence of infectious diseases.
[12]When the first unit has been tested but any unit collected within 30 days after the first collection has not been tested.
[13]Labeling of Recovered Plasma shall conform to 21 CFR 606.121(e)(4) and 21 CFR 610.40(h)(2)(ii).

Reference Standard 5.1.8A—Requirements for Storage, Transportation, and Expiration

Item No.	Component	Storage	Transport	Expiration[1]	Additional Criteria
Whole Blood Components					
1	Whole Blood	1-6 C. If intended for room temperature components, then store at 1-6 C within 8 hours after collection	Cooling toward 1-10 C. If intended for room temperature components, cooling toward 20-24 C	ACD/CPD/CP2D: 21 days CPDA-1: 35 days	
2	Whole Blood Irradiated	1-6 C	1-10 C	Original expiration or 28 days from date of irradiation, whichever is sooner	
Red Blood Cell Components					
3	Red Blood Cells (RBCs)	1-6 C	1-10 C	ACD/CPD/CP2D: 21 days CPDA-1: 35 days Additive solution: 42 days Open system: 24 hours	

(Continued)

Reference Standard 5.1.8A—Requirements for Storage, Transportation, and Expiration (Continued)

Item No.	Component	Storage	Transport	Expiration[1]	Additional Criteria
4	Deglycerolized RBCs	1-6 C	1-10 C	Open system: 24 hours / Closed system: 14 days or as FDA approved	
5	Frozen RBCs 40% Glycerol	≤-65 C if 40% glycerol or as FDA approved	Maintain frozen state	10 years (A policy shall be developed if rare frozen units are to be retained beyond this time)	Frozen within 6 days of collection unless rejuvenated / Frozen before Red Blood Cell expiration if rare unit
6	RBCs Irradiated	1-6 C	1-10 C	Original expiration or 28 days from date of irradiation, whichever is sooner	
7	RBCs Leukocytes Reduced	1-6 C	1-10 C	ACD/CPD/CP2D: 21 days / CPDA-1: 35 days / Additive solution: 42 days / Open system: 24 hours	

8	Rejuvenated RBCs	1-6 C	1-10 C	CPD, CPDA-1: 24 hours	AS-1: freeze after rejuvenation
9	Deglycerolized Rejuvenated RBCs	1-6 C	1-10 C	24 hours or as approved by FDA	
10	Frozen Rejuvenated RBCs	≤-65 C	Maintain frozen state	CPD, CPDA-1: 10 years AS-1: 3 years (A policy shall be developed if rare frozen units are to be retained beyond this time)	
11	Washed RBCs	1-6 C	1-10 C	24 hours	
12	Apheresis RBCs	1-6 C	1-10 C	CPDA-1: 35 days Additive solution: 42 days Open system: 24 hours	
13	Apheresis RBCs Leukocytes Reduced	1-6 C	1-10 C	CPDA-1: 35 days Additive solution: 42 days Open system: 24 hours	
14	Platelets	20-24 C with continuous gentle agitation	As close as possible to 20-24 C^2	24 hours to 5 days, depending on collection system	Maximum time without agitation: 24 hours

(Continued)

Reference Standard 5.1.8A—Requirements for Storage, Transportation, and Expiration (Continued)

Item No.	Component	Storage	Transport	Expiration[1]	Additional Criteria
Platelet Components					
15	Platelets—Irradiated	20-24 C with continuous gentle agitation	As close as possible to 20-24 C[2]	No change from original expiration date	Maximum time without agitation: 24 hours
16	Platelets—Leukocytes Reduced	20-24 C with continuous gentle agitation	As close as possible to 20-24 C[2]	Open system: 4 hours Closed system: No change in expiration	Maximum time without agitation: 24 hours
17	Pooled Platelets Leukocytes Reduced	20-24 C with continuous gentle agitation	As close as possible to 20-24 C[2]	4 hours after pooling or 5 days following collection of the oldest unit in the pool[3]	Maximum time without agitation: 24 hours
18	Pooled Platelets (in open system)	20-24 C with continuous gentle agitation	As close as possible to 20-24 C[2]	Open system: 4 hours	
19	Apheresis Platelets	20-24 C with continuous gentle agitation	As close as possible to 20-24 C[2]	24 hours or 5 days, depending on collection system	Maximum time without agitation: 24 hours
20	Apheresis Platelets Irradiated	20-24 C with continuous gentle agitation	As close as possible to 20-24 C[2]	No change from original expiration date	Maximum time without agitation: 24 hours

No.	Component	Storage Temperature	Transport Temperature	Expiration/Storage Period	Notes
21	Apheresis Platelets Leukocytes Reduced	20-24 C with continuous gentle agitation	As close as possible to 20-24 C²	Open system: within 4 hours of opening the system Closed system: 5 days	Maximum time without agitation: 24 hours
22	Apheresis Platelets Platelet Additive Solution Added Leukocytes Reduced	20-24 C with continuous gentle agitation	As close as possible to 20-24 C²	5 days	Maximum time without agitation: 24 hours
Granulocyte Components					
23	Apheresis Granulocytes	20-24 C	As close as possible to 20-24 C	24 hours	Transfuse as soon as possible; Standard 5.28.10 applies
24	Apheresis Granulocytes Irradiated	20-24 C	As close as possible to 20-24 C	No change from original expiration date	Transfuse as soon as possible; Standard 5.28.10 applies
25	Cryoprecipitated AHF	≤−18 C	Maintain frozen state	12 months from original collection	Thaw the FFP at 1-6 C Place cryoprecipitate in the freezer within 1 hour after removal from refrigerated centrifuge

(Continued)

Reference Standard 5.1.8A—Requirements for Storage, Transportation, and Expiration (Continued)

Item No.	Component	Storage	Transport	Expiration[1]	Additional Criteria
Plasma Components					
26	Cryoprecipitated AHF (after thawing)	20-24 C	As close as possible to 20-24 C	Single unit: 6 hours	Thaw at 30-37 C
27	Pooled Cryoprecipitated AHF (pooled before freezing)	≤-18C	Maintain frozen state	12 months from earliest date of collection of product in pool	Thaw the FFP at 1-6 C Place cryoprecipitate in the freezer within 1 hour after removal from refrigerated centrifuge
28	Pooled Cryoprecipitated AHF (after thawing)	20-24 C	As close as possible to 20-24 C	Pooled in an open system: 4 hours. If pooled using a sterile connection device: 6 hours	Thaw at 30-37 C
29	Fresh Frozen Plasma (FFP)[5]	≤-18 C or ≤-65 C	Maintain frozen state	≤-18 C: 12 months from collection; ≤-65 C: 7 years from collection	Placed in freezer within 8 hours of collection or as stated in FDA-cleared operator's manuals/package inserts

Storage at ≤–65 requires FDA approval if product is stored for longer than 12 months

#	Component	Storage	Transport	Expiration	Notes
30	FFP (after thawing)[5]	1-6 C	1-10 C	If issued as FFP: 24 hours	Thaw at 30-37 C or using an FDA-cleared device
31	Plasma Frozen Within 24 Hours After Phlebotomy (PF24)[5]	≤–18 C	Maintain frozen state	12 months from collection	
32	Plasma Frozen Within 24 Hours After Phlebotomy (after thawing)[5]	1-6 C	1-10 C	If issued as PF24: 24 hours	Thaw at 30-37 C or using an FDA-cleared device
33	Plasma Frozen Within 24 Hours After Phlebotomy Held At Room Temperature Up To 24 Hours After Phlebotomy (PF24RT24)	≤–18 C or colder	Maintain frozen state	12 months from collection	

(Continued)

Reference Standard 5.1.8A—Requirements for Storage, Transportation, and Expiration (Continued)

Item No.	Component	Storage	Transport	Expiration[1]	Additional Criteria
34	Plasma Frozen Within 24 Hours After Phlebotomy Held At Room Temperature Up To 24 Hours After Phlebotomy (after thawing)	1-6 C	1-10 C	If issued as PF24RT24: 24 hours	Thaw at 30-37 C or using an FDA-cleared device
35	Thawed Plasma[5]	1-6 C	1-10 C	5 days from date product was thawed or original expiration, whichever is sooner	Shall have been collected and processed in a closed system
36	Plasma Cryoprecipitate Reduced	≤-18 C	Maintain frozen state	12 months from collection	
37	Plasma Cryoprecipitate Reduced (after thawing)	1-6 C	1-10 C	If issued as Plasma Cryoprecipitate Reduced: 24 hours	Thaw at 30-37 C
38	Thawed Plasma Cryoprecipitate Reduced	1-6 C	1-10 C	If issued as Thawed Plasma Cryoprecipitate Reduced: 5 days from date product was thawed or original expiration, whichever is sooner	Shall have been collected and processed in a closed system

No.	Component				
39	Liquid Plasma	1-6 C	1-10 C	5 days after expiration of Whole Blood	21 CFR 610.53(c) applies
40	Recovered Plasma, liquid or frozen	Refer to short supply agreement	Refer to short supply agreement	Refer to short supply agreement	Requires a short sup-ply agreement[4]
Tissue and Derivatives					
41	Tissue	Conform to source facility's written instructions	Conform to source facility's written instructions	Conform to source facility's written instructions	21 CFR 1271.3(b), 1271.3(bb), and 21 CFR 1271.15(d) apply
42	Derivatives	Conform to manufac-turer's written instructions	Conform to manufac-turer's written instructions	Conform to manufac-turer's written instructions	

[1]If the seal is broken during processing, components stored at 1 to 6 C shall have an expiration time of 24 hours, and components stored at 20 to 24 C shall have an expiration time of 4 hours, unless otherwise indicated. This expiration shall not exceed the original expiration date or time.
[2]21 CFR 600.15(a).
[3]Storage beyond 4 hours requires an FDA-cleared system.
[4]21 CFR 601.22.
[5]These lines could apply to apheresis plasma or whole-blood-derived plasma.

Reference Standard 5.4.1A—Requirements for Allogeneic Donor Qualification*

Category	Criteria/Description/Examples	Deferral Period
1) Age	• Conform to applicable state law or • ≥16 years	
2) Whole Blood Volume Collected	• Maximum of 10.5 mL/kg of donor weight, including samples	
3) Donation Interval	• 8 weeks after whole blood donation (Standards 5.5.1-5.5.4 and 5.6.7.1 apply) • 16 weeks after 2-unit Red Blood Cell collection • 4 weeks after infrequent plasmapheresis • ≥2 days after plasma-, platelet-, or leukapheresis	
4) Temperature	• ≤37.5 C (99.5 F) if measured orally, or equivalent if measured by another method	
5) Hemoglobin/Hematocrit	• ≥12.5 g/dL or ≥38%; blood obtained by earlobe puncture shall not be used for this determination • For double Red Blood Cell collections, follow instrument operator's manual	
6) Drug Therapy†	• Generic medication name [example of trade name(s)] • Finasteride (eg, Proscar, Propecia) • Isotretinoin (eg, Absorica, Accutane, Amnesteem, Claravis, Myorisan, Sotret, Zenatane) • Dutasteride (eg, Avodart, Jaylyn) • Acitretin (eg, Soriatane) • Etretinate (eg, Tegison)	 1 month after last dose 6 months after last dose 3 years after last dose Permanent

• Bovine insulin manufactured in the UK	Indefinite
• Medications that irreversibly inhibit platelet function preclude use of the donor as sole source of platelets	
a. Aspirin, aspirin-containing medications and piroxicam (eg, Feldene)	2 full days (>48 hours) after last dose
b. Prasugrel (Effient) and ticagrelor (Brilinta)	7 days
c. Clopidogrel (eg, Plavix) and ticlopidine (eg, Ticlid)	14 days after last dose
• Warfarin (eg, Coumadin, Warfilone, Jantoven)	For plasma products for transfusion: 1 week (7 days) after last dose
• Heparin and derivatives	For plasma products for transfusion: 1 week (7 days) after last dose or as defined by the facility's medical director
• Direct thrombin inhibitors (eg, dabigatran)	
• Direct Xa inhibitors (eg, rivaroxaban)	
• Receipt of Hepatitis B Immune Globulin	12 months
• Other medications, such as antibiotics	As defined by the facility's medical director
7) Medical History and General Health	• The prospective donor shall appear to be in good health and shall be free of major organ disease (eg, heart, liver, lungs), cancer, or abnormal bleeding tendency, unless determined suitable by the medical director
	• The venipuncture site shall be evaluated for lesions on the skin
	• The venipuncture site shall be free from infectious skin disease and any disease that might create a risk of contaminating the blood
	• Family history of Creutzfeldt-Jakob disease (CJD)[1] — Indefinite deferral for risk of CJD

(Continued)

Reference Standard 5.4.1A—Requirements for Allogeneic Donor Qualification[*] (Continued)

Category	Criteria/Description/Examples	Deferral Period
8) Pregnancy	• Defer if pregnant within the last 6 weeks	
9) Receipt of Blood, Blood Component, or Human Tissue	• Receipt of dura mater or pituitary growth hormone of human origin	Indefinite
	• Receipt of blood, components, human tissue, or plasma-derived clotting factor concentrates	12 months
10) Immunizations and -Vaccinations	• Receipt of toxoids, or synthetic or killed viral, bacterial, or rickettsial vaccines if donor is symptom-free and afebrile [Anthrax, Cholera, Diphtheria, Hepatitis A, Hepatitis B, Influenza, Lyme disease, Paratyphoid, Pertussis, Plague, Pneumococcal polysaccharide, Polio (Salk/injection), Rabies, Rocky Mountain spotted fever, Tetanus, Typhoid (by injection)]	None
	• Receipt of recombinant vaccine (eg, HPV vaccine)	
	• Receipt of intranasal live attenuated flu vaccine	
	• Receipt of live attenuated viral and bacterial vaccines [Measles (rubeola), Mumps, Polio (Sabin/oral), Typhoid (oral), Yellow fever]	2 weeks
	• Receipt of live attenuated viral and bacterial vaccines [German measles (rubella), chicken pox/shingles (varicella zoster)]	4 weeks
	• Smallpox[2]	Refer to FDA Guidance

• Receipt of other vaccines, including unlicensed vaccines	12 months unless otherwise indicated by medical director
11) Infectious Diseases	
• History of viral hepatitis after 11th birthday	Indefinite
• Confirmed positive test for HBsAg[3]	Permanent
• Repeatedly reactive test for anti-HBc on more than one occasion[4]	Indefinite
• Positive HBV NAT result[5]	
• Repeatedly reactive test for anti-HTLV on more than one occasion	Indefinite[6]
• Present or past clinical or laboratory evidence of infection with HIV, HCV, HTLV, or *T. cruzi* or as excluded by current FDA regulations and recommendations for the prevention of HIV transmission by blood and components	Indefinite
• A history of babesiosis	Indefinite
• Evidence or obvious stigmata of parenteral drug use	Indefinite
• Use of a needle to administer nonprescription drugs	Indefinite
• Mucous membrane exposure to blood	12 months
• Nonsterile skin penetration with instruments or equipment contaminated with blood or body fluids other than the donor's own	12 months
• Includes tattoos or permanent make-up unless applied by a state regulated entity with sterile needles and ink that has not been reused	

(Continued)

63

Reference Standard 5.4.1A—Requirements for Allogeneic Donor Qualification* (Continued)

Category	Criteria/Description/Examples	Deferral Period
	• Sexual contact or lived with an individual who: a. Has acute or chronic hepatitis B (positive HBsAg test, HBV NAT)	12 months
	b. Has symptomatic hepatitis C	
	c. Is symptomatic for any other viral hepatitis	
	• Sexual contact with an individual with HIV infection or at high risk of HIV infection[7,8]	12 months or as recommended by FDA
	• Incarceration in a correctional institution (including juvenile detention, lockup, jail, or prison) for more than 72 consecutive hours	12 months
	• Syphilis or gonorrhea[9] a. Following the diagnosis of syphilis or gonorrhea. Must have completed treatment	12 months (in accordance with FDA Guidance)
	b. Donor who has a reactive screening test for syphilis where no confirmatory testing was performed	
	c. A confirmed positive test for syphilis (FDA reentry protocol applies)	
	• West Nile virus	In accordance with FDA Guidance[10]

- Malaria[11]

These deferral periods apply in nonendemic countries, irrespective of the receipt of antimalarial prophylaxis:

a. Prospective donors who have had a diagnosis of malaria

   a. 3 years after becoming asymptomatic

b. Individuals who have lived longer than 5 consecutive years in countries considered malaria-endemic by the Malarial Branch, Centers for Disease Control and Prevention, US Department of Health and Human Services

   b. 3 years after departure from malaria-endemic country(ies) lived in

c. Individuals who have lived longer than 5 consecutive years in countries considered malaria-endemic by the Malarial Branch, Centers for Disease Control and Prevention, US Department of Health and Human Services who have traveled to an area where malaria is endemic before living at least 3 consecutive years in nonendemic country(ies)

   c. 3 years after departure from malaria-endemic area(s) traveled to

d. Individuals who either:

  i. Traveled to an area where malaria is endemic

  ii. Lived longer than 5 consecutive years in countries considered malaria-endemic by the Malarial Branch, Centers for Disease Control and Prevention, US Department of Health and Human Services who have traveled to an area where malaria is endemic after having lived at least 3 consecutive years in nonendemic country(ies)[12]

   d. Defer for 12 months after departure from malaria-endemic area(s) traveled to

(Continued)

Reference Standard 5.4.1A—Requirements for Allogeneic Donor Qualification* (Continued)

Category	Criteria/Description/Examples	Deferral Period
12) Travel	• The prospective donor's travel history shall be evaluated for potential risks[1,8,11,12]	
	• Donors recommended for deferral for risk of vCJD, as defined in most recent FDA Guidance[1]	Indefinite

*For blood pressure, see 21 CFR 640.3(b)(2).

†Medication Deferral List current version at http://www.aabb.org/resources/donation/questionnaires/Pages/dhqaabb.aspx.

[1]FDA Guidance for Industry: Revised Preventive Measures to Reduce the Possible Risk of Transmission of Creutzfeldt-Jakob Disease (CJD) and Variant Creutzfeldt-Jakob Disease (vCJD) by Blood and Blood Products, May 27, 2010.

[2]FDA Guidance for Industry: Recommendations for Deferral of Donors and Quarantine and Retrieval of Blood and Blood Products in Recent Recipients of Smallpox Vaccine (Vaccinia Virus) and Certain Contacts of Smallpox Vaccine Recipients, December 30, 2002.

[3]FDA Memorandum: Recommendations for the Management of Donors and Units that Are Initially Reactive for Hepatitis B Surface Antigen, December 2, 1987.

FDA Guidance for Industry: Requalification Method for Reentry of Donors Who Test Hepatitis B Surface Antigen (HBsAg) Positive Following a Recent Vaccination against Hepatitis B Virus Infection, November 2011.

[4]FDA Memorandum to All Registered Blood Establishments, FDA Recommendations Concerning Testing for Antibody to Hepatitis B Core Antigen (Anti-HBc), September 10, 1991.

FDA Guidance for Industry: Requalification Method for Reentry of Blood Donors Deferred Because of Reactive Test Results for Antibody to Hepatitis B Core Antigen (Anti-HBc), May 30, 2010.

[5]FDA Guidance for Industry: Use of Nucleic Acid Tests on Pooled and Individual Samples from Donors of Whole Blood and Blood Components, Including Source Plasma, to Reduce the Risk of Transmission of Hepatitis B Virus, October 2012.

[6]FDA Guidance for Industry: Donor Screening for Antibodies to HTLV-II, August 15, 1997.

[7]FDA Memorandum: Revised Recommendation for the Prevention of Human Immunodeficiency Virus (HIV) Transmission by Blood and Blood Products, April 23, 1992.

[8] FDA Guidance for Industry: Recommendations for Management of Donors at Increased Risk for Human Immunodeficiency Virus Type I (HIV) Group O Infection, August 2009.

[9] FDA Memorandum to All Registered Blood Establishments: Clarification of FDA Recommendations for Donor Deferral and Product Distribution Based on the Results of Syphilis Testing, December 12, 1991.

[10] FDA Guidance for Industry: Use of Nucleic Acid Tests to Reduce the Risk of Transmission of West Nile Virus from Donors of Whole Blood and Blood Components Intended for Transfusion, November 6, 2009.

[11] FDA Memorandum to All Registered Blood Establishments: Recommendations for Deferral of Donors for Malaria Risk, July 26, 1994. FDA Memorandum to All Registered Blood Establishments: Recommendations for the Deferral of Current and Recent Inmates of Correctional Institutions as Donors of Whole Blood, Blood Components, Source Leukocytes and Source Plasma, June 8, 1995.

[12] www.cdc.gov/travel.

6. DOCUMENTS AND RECORDS

6.0 Documents and Records

The blood bank or transfusion service shall have policies, processes, and procedures to ensure that documents are identified, reviewed, approved, and retained and that records are created, stored, and archived in accordance with record retention policies.

6.1 Documents

The blood bank or transfusion service shall have a process for document control that includes the following elements:

6.1.1
Master list(s) of documents, including policies, processes, procedures, labels, and forms that relate to the requirements of these *BBTS Standards*.

6.1.2
Use of standardized formats for all policies, processes, procedures, and forms. Additional procedures (such as those in an operator's manual or published in the AABB *Technical Manual*) may be incorporated by reference.

6.1.3
Review and approval of new and revised documents before use.

6.1.4
Review of each policy, process, and procedure shall be performed by an authorized individual at a minimum every 2 years.

6.1.5
Use of only current and valid documents. Appropriate and applicable documents shall be available at all locations where activities essential to meeting the requirements of these *BBTS Standards* are performed.

6.1.6
Identification and appropriate archival of obsolete documents.

6.1.7
Storage in a manner that preserves legibility and protects from accidental or unauthorized access, destruction, or modification.

6.2 Records

The blood bank or transfusion service shall ensure identification, collection, indexing, access, filing, storage, and disposition of records as required by Reference Standards 6.2A through 6.2E, Retention of Records.

6.2.1 Facility Records

Records shall be complete, retrievable in a period appropriate to the circumstances, and protected from accidental or unauthorized destruction or modification.

6.2.1.1 Records shall be legible and indelible.

6.2.1.2 Copies

Before the destruction of the original records, the blood bank or transfusion service shall have a process to ensure that copies of records are:
1) Verified as containing the original content.
2) Legible, complete, and accessible.

6.2.2 A system designed to prevent unauthorized access and ensure confidentiality of records shall be established and followed.

6.2.3 The record system shall make it possible to trace any unit of blood, blood component, tissue, or derivative from its source to final disposition; to review the records applying to the specific component; and to investigate adverse events manifested by the recipient.

6.2.4 Records shall be created and maintained to include:
1) Critical activities performed.
2) The individual who performed the activity.
3) When the activity was performed.
4) Results obtained.
5) Method(s) used (when more than one method is in use).
6) Equipment used.
7) Critical materials used.
8) The facility where the activity was performed.

6.2.4.1 The system shall ensure that the donor and patient identifiers are unique.

6.2.5 Records shall be created concurrently with performance of each critical activity.

6.2.5.1 The actual result of each test performed shall be recorded immediately, and the final interpretation shall be recorded upon completion of testing.

6.2.6 Changes to Records
Changes to records shall be controlled.

6.2.6.1 The date of changes and the identity of the individual who changed the record shall be documented, and this information shall be maintained for the retention period of the original record.

6.2.6.2 Record changes shall not obscure previously recorded information.

6.2.6.3 Changes to records (including electronic records) shall be verified for accuracy and completeness.

6.2.7 Electronic Records
There shall be processes and procedures to support the management of computer systems.

6.2.7.1 There shall be a process in place for routine backup of all critical data.

6.2.7.1.1 Procedures shall be in place to ensure that data are retrievable and usable.

6.2.7.1.2 Backup data shall be stored in an off-site location.

6.2.8 Storage of Records
Records shall be stored to:
1) Preserve record legibility and integrity for the entire retention period.
2) Protect from accidental or unauthorized access, destruction, or modification.
3) Allow retrieval.

6.2.9 Destruction of Records
Destruction of records shall be conducted in a manner that protects the confidential content of the records.

Reference Standard 6.2A—Retention of Donor/Unit Records

Item No.	Standard	Record to Be Maintained	Minimum Retention Time (in years)[1,2]
1	4.3	Inspection of incoming blood and blood components	10
2	5.1.6.1	Identification of individuals performing each significant step in collection, processing, compatibility testing, and transportation of blood and blood components	10
3	5.1.6.2	Traceability of blood, blood components, tissue, derivatives, and critical materials	10
4	5.1.6.5	Source to final disposition of each unit of blood or blood component and, if issued by the facility for transfusion, identification of the recipient	10
5	5.1.6.5.1 5.1.6.5.2	Unique identification of each unit	10
6	5.2.1 #6	Donor acknowledgment that educational materials have been read	10
7	5.2.2	Parental permission for donation	10
8	5.2.3	Consent of donors	10
9	5.2.4	Notification to donor of significant abnormal findings	10
10	5.2.4	Donors placed on permanent deferral, and indefinite deferral for protection of recipient	Indefinite
11	5.4.1 5.4.2	Donor information, including address, medical history, physical examination, health history, or other conditions thought to compromise suitability of blood or blood component	10
12	5.4.4.1	A medical order from the patient's physician is required to collect blood for autologous use	10
13	5.5.3.4	Platelet count for frequent plateletpheresis donors	10

(Continued)

Reference Standard 6.2A—Retention of Donor/Unit Records (Continued)

Item No.	Standard	Record to Be Maintained	Minimum Retention Time (in years)[1,2]
14	5.6.6.2	Cytapheresis record, including anticoagulant drugs given, duration of procedure, volume of components, drugs used, lot number of disposables, and replacement fluids	10
15	5.6.6.2.1	Maximal cumulative dose of sedimenting agent administered to donor in a given time	10
16	5.7.2.1	Inspection of weld for completeness and identification numbers of blood or blood components and of lot numbers of disposables used during component preparation	10
17	5.7.3.2.1	Verification of irradiation dose delivery	10
18	5.7.3.3	Donation identification number and collecting facility for each unit in pooled components	10
19	5.7.4	Preparation of specific components	10
20	5.8.1 5.8.2	ABO group and Rh type for all collections	10
21	5.8.3.1	Allogeneic donor testing to detect unexpected antibodies to red cell antigens	10
22	5.8.3.3	Control system results appropriate to the method of testing	10
23	5.8.5	Interpretations of disease marker testing for allogeneic testing	10
24	5.8.5.1	Distribution or issue of units before completion of tests	10
25	5.8.7	Quarantine of units from prior collections when a repeat donor has a reactive disease marker screening test	10
26	5.9.1	Final review of records relating to testing and acceptability criteria	10
27	5.9.4	Review of donor records to ensure any units from an ineligible donor are quarantined	10

Reference Standard 6.2A—Retention of Donor/Unit Records (Continued)

Item No.	Standard	Record to Be Maintained	Minimum Retention Time (in years)[1,2]
28	5.12	Serologic confirmation of donor blood ABO/Rh	10
29	5.12.1	Reporting and resolution of ABO/Rh labeling discrepancies to collecting facility	10
30	5.26	If a unit is returned for reissue, confirmation that the tubing identification number on reattached segments is identical and confirmation that the blood or blood components have been inspected and are acceptable	10
31	5.27	A signed statement from the requesting physician indicating that the clinical situation was sufficiently urgent to require release of blood before completion of compatibility testing or infectious disease testing	10
32	7.1.4	Blood and blood components that are determined after release not to conform to specified requirements	10
33	7.3	Adverse events related to donation	10
34	7.4.2.4	Notification by consignee of a transfusion fatality or other serious adverse event	10
35	7.4.5.2	Collection facility's investigation of transmissible diseases	10
36	7.4.6	Look-back investigation	10

[1]Applicable state or local law may exceed this period.
[2]21 CFR 606.160(d).

Reference Standard 6.2B—Retention of Patient Records

Item No.	Standard	Record to Be Maintained	Minimum Retention Time (in Years)[1,2]
1	5.1.6.5	Source to final disposition of each unit of blood or blood component and, if issued by the facility for transfusion, identification of the recipient	10
2	5.6.7	Therapeutic apheresis: physician request, patient identification, diagnosis, type of therapeutic procedure performed, method used, vital signs before and after the procedure, extracorporeal blood volume if applicable, nature and volume of component removed, nature and volume of replacement fluids, any occurrence of adverse events, and medication administered Therapeutic phlebotomy: physician, request, patient identification, diagnosis, vital signs before the procedure, volume removed, and any occurrence of adverse events	5
3	5.11.1	Requests for blood and blood components	5
4	5.11.1.1	Order for blood, blood components, tests, and derivatives	5
5	5.14.1 5.14.2	Test results and interpretation of patient's ABO group and Rh type	10
6	5.14.3	Patient testing to detect unexpected antibodies to red cell antigens	10
7	5.14.3.1	Additional testing to detect clinically significant antibodies	10
8	5.14.3.4	Control system results appropriate to the method of testing	10
9	5.14.4	Pretransfusion testing for autologous transfusion	10
10	5.14.5(1)	ABO group and Rh type	10
11	5.14.5 (2,3,4,5)	Difficulty in blood typing, clinically significant antibodies, significant adverse events to transfusion, and special transfusion requirements	Indefinite

Reference Standard 6.2B–Retention of Patient Records (Continued)

Item No.	Standard	Record to Be Maintained	Minimum Retention Time (in Years)[1,2]
12	5.16.1	Test results and interpretation of serologic cross-match	10
13	5.16.1.1	Detection of ABO incompatibility when no clinically significant antibodies are detected	10
14	5.16.2.2	Two determinations of the recipient's ABO group	10
15	5.16.2.3	Computer detection of ABO incompatibility	10
16	5.17.1	ABO/Rh of neonatal recipients	10
17	5.17.1.3	Selection of compatible units when initial antibody screen for neonates demonstrates clinically significant antibodies	10
18	5.17.2	Testing of the neonate's serum or plasma for anti-A or anti-B if a non-group-O neonate is to receive non-group-O Red Blood Cells that are not compatible with the maternal ABO group	10
19	5.18	Intrauterine Transfusion Policy	10
20	5.19.3.1	Irradiation of cellular components, if applicable	10
21	5.22	Final inspection of blood and blood components before issue; if the container is not intact or components are abnormal in appearance, maintain record of medical director approval	10
22	5.23	Verification at issue of: 1. The intended recipient's two independent identifiers, ABO group, and Rh type 2. The donation identification number, the donor ABO group, and, if required, the Rh type 3. The interpretation of crossmatch tests, if performed 4. Special transfusion requirements, if applicable	10

(Continued)

Reference Standard 6.2B—Retention of Patient Records (Continued)

Item No.	Standard	Record to Be Maintained	Minimum Retention Time (in Years)[1,2]
22 (Cont.)		5. The expiration date and, if applicable, time 6. The date and time of issue 7. Personnel issuing and accepting blood components	
23	5.27.5	A signed statement from the requesting physician indicating that the clinical situation was sufficiently urgent to require release of blood before completion of compatibility testing or infectious disease testing	10
24	5.27.5.1	Notification of abnormal test results	10
25	5.28.1	Recipient consent	5
26	5.28.3	Verification of the following information before transfusion: The intended recipient's two independent identifiers, ABO group, and Rh type The donation identification number, the donor ABO group, and, if required, the Rh type The interpretation of crossmatch tests, if performed Special transfusion requirements are met, when applicable The expiration date (or time) of the unit and that it has not expired	5
27	5.28.4	Verification of patient identification before transfusion	5
28	5.29.1, 7.4	Patient's medical record: transfusion order, documentation of patient consent, component name, donation identification number, date and time of transfusion, pre- and posttransfusion vital signs, the amount transfused, identification of the transfusionist, and, if applicable, transfusion-related adverse events	5

Reference Standard 6.2B–Retention of Patient Records (Continued)

Item No.	Standard	Record to Be Maintained	Minimum Retention Time (in Years)[1,2]
29	7.4.1.2	Immediate evaluation of suspected transfusion reactions	10
30	7.4.2 7.4.2.1	Laboratory evaluation and review of clerical information related to suspected hemolytic reactions	10
31	7.4.2.3	Interpretation of the evaluation of suspected immediate transfusion adverse events	10
32	7.4.3	Evaluation and interpretation of delayed transfusion adverse events	10
33	7.4.6	Look-back to identify recipients who may have been infected with HCV or HIV	10

[1]Applicable state or local law may exceed this period.
[2]21 CFR 606.160(d).

Reference Standard 6.2C–Retention of Other Documents and Records

Item No.	Standard	Record to Be Maintained	Minimum Retention Time (in years)[1,2]
1	1.2.2	Management review of effectiveness of the quality system	5
2	1.3.2	Exceptions to policies, processes, and procedures	10
3	1.4.1	Emergency operation plan tested at defined intervals	2
4	2.1	Job descriptions	5
5	2.1.1	Qualification of personnel performing critical tasks	5
6	2.1.2	Training records of personnel	5
7	2.1.3	Evaluations of competence of personnel	5
8	2.1.4	Personnel records of each employee	5
9	2.1.4.1	Records of names, signatures, initials or identification codes, and inclusive dates of employment for personnel who perform or review critical tasks	10
10	3.2	Equipment qualification	10 after retirement of the equipment
11	3.4	Unique identification of equipment	5
12	3.5	Monitoring and maintenance of equipment	10 after retirement of the equipment
13	3.6.2	Temperature monitoring of refrigerators, freezers, and platelet incubators	10
14	3.6.3	Monitoring of liquid nitrogen levels or temperature	10
15	3.9	Implementation and modification of software, hardware, or databases	2 after retirement of the system
16	3.9.1	Validation of system software, hardware, databases, user-defined tables, electronic data transfer, and/or electronic data receipt	2 after retirement of the system

Reference Standard 6.2C—Retention of Other Documents and Records (Continued)

Item No.	Standard	Record to Be Maintained	Minimum Retention Time (in years)[1,2]
16 (Cont.)		Fulfillment of applicable life-cycle requirements	
		Numerical designation of system versions, if applicable, with inclusive dates of use	
		Monitoring of data integrity for critical data elements	
17	4.1	Evaluation and participation in selection of suppliers	5
18	4.2	Agreements	5
19	4.2.1	Agreement review	5
20	4.2.2	Agreements concerning activities involving more than one facility	5
21	4.3	Inspection of incoming critical materials and containers	10
22	4.3.2.1	Incoming containers, solutions, and reagents meet or exceed applicable FDA criteria	10
23	5.1.1	Validation of new or changed processes and procedures	5
24	5.1.2	Participation in proficiency testing program	5
25	5.1.3	Quality control records and review of quality control results for reagents, equipment, and methods	10
26	5.1.4.1	Reagents prepared by facility meet or exceed FDA criteria	10
27	5.1.8.1.3	Records of storage temperatures for blood products	10
28	5.1.8.1.3.1	Ambient temperature recorded every 4 hours when components are stored in open storage area	10

(Continued)

Reference Standard 6.2C–Retention of Other Documents and Records (Continued)

Item No.	Standard	Record to Be Maintained	Minimum Retention Time (in years)[1,2]
29	5.1.8.2	Inspection before shipping	10
30	5.1.8.2.1	Container qualification and process validation records	10
31	5.28.1	Participation in development of policies, processes, and procedures regarding recipient consent for transfusion	5
32	6.1.3	Review and approval of new and revised documents before use	5
33	6.1.4	Biennial review of policies, processes, and procedures	5
34	6.1.6	Identification and appropriate archival of obsolete documents	5
35	7.0 7.1	Description and evaluation of nonconforming blood, blood components, tissue, derivatives, critical materials, and services	10
36	7.1.4	Nature of nonconformances discovered after release and subsequent actions taken, including acceptance for use	10
37	7.1.4.1	Disposition of nonconforming products	10
38	7.2	Fatality reports	10
39	7.4.5.1	Transfusion service evaluation and reporting of transmissible diseases	10
40	8.1.2	Review of assessment results	5
41	8.2	Peer-review assessment of blood utilization	5
42	9.0	Implementation of changes to policies, processes, and procedures resulting from corrective and preventive action	5
43	9.1	Corrective action	5
44	9.2	Preventive action	5

Reference Standard 6.2C—Retention of Other Documents and Records (Continued)

Item No.	Standard	Record to Be Maintained	Minimum Retention Time (in years)[1,2]
45	10.2	Monitoring of biological, chemical, and radiation safety	5
46	10.3	Appropriate discard of blood and blood components	10

[1]Applicable state or local law may exceed this period.
[2]21 CFR 606.160(d).

Reference Standard 6.2D—Retention of Tissue Records

Item No.	Standard	Record to Be Maintained	Minimum Retention Time (in years)[1]
1	4.3	Inspection of incoming tissue upon receipt	10
2	5.1.6.2	Traceability of tissue to final disposition	10
3	5.11.1	Requests for tissue	10
4	5.20	Preparation of tissue including: 1. Type of tissue 2. Numeric or alphanumeric identifier 3. Quantity 4. Expiration date and, if applicable, time 5. Personnel who prepared tissue	10
5	5.24	Issue of tissue, including: 1. The manufacturer's package insert documents are present and are issued 2. Product quantity and name matches request 3. Final inspection 4. Personnel dispensing tissue 5. Personnel accepting tissue for use 6. If issued for a particular patient, the intended recipient's two independent identifiers 7. The date and time of issue	10
6	5.26	If a tissue is returned for reissue, confirmation that the container closure has not been disturbed and confirmation that the tissue is suitable for reissue	10
7	5.29.2	Patient's medical record for receipt of tissue to include type of tissue, numeric or alphanumeric identifier, quantity, expiration date and date of use, personnel using the tissue, and, if applicable, related adverse events	10 beyond the date of final disposition
8	7.1	Identification of nonconforming tissue	10

Reference Standard 6.2D—Retention of Tissue Records (Continued)

Item No.	Standard	Record to Be Maintained	Minimum Retention Time (in years)[1]
9	7.4.4	Investigation of adverse effects, disease transmission, or other suspected adverse events of tissue use and reporting of such cases to the source facility, manufacturer, and outside agencies as required	10
10	10.3	Appropriate discard of tissue	10

[1]Applicable state or local law may exceed this period.

Reference Standard 6.2E—Retention of Derivative Records

Item No.	Standard	Record to Be Maintained	Minimum Retention Time (in years)[1]
1	4.3	Inspection of incoming derivatives upon receipt	10
2	5.1.6.2	Traceability of derivatives to final disposition	10
3	5.11.1	Requests for derivatives	10
4	5.21	Preparation of derivatives to include: 1. Type of derivative 2. Lot number 3. Quantity 4. Expiration date and, if applicable, time 5. Personnel who prepared the derivative	10
5	5.24	Issue of derivatives, including: 1. The manufacturer's package insert documents are present and are issued 2. Product quantity and name matches request 3. Final inspection 4. Personnel dispensing derivative 5. Personnel accepting derivative for use 6. If issued for a particular patient, the intended recipient's two independent identifiers 7. The date and time of issue	10
6	5.26	If a derivative is returned for reissue, confirmation that the container closure has not been disturbed and confirmation that the derivative is suitable for reissue	10

Reference Standard 6.2E—Retention of Derivative Records (Continued)

Item No.	Standard	Record to Be Maintained	Minimum Retention Time (in years)[1]
7	5.29.3	Patient's medical record for receipt of derivatives to include product name, lot number, quantity, administration date and time, individuals administering the derivative, and, if applicable, related adverse events	10 beyond the date of distribution, date of infusion, date of disposition, or date of expiration, whichever is the latest date
8	7.1	Identification of nonconforming derivatives	10
9	7.4.4	Investigation of adverse effects, disease transmission, or other suspected adverse events of derivative use and reporting of such cases to the source facility, manufacturer, and outside agencies as required	10
10	10.3	Appropriate discard of derivatives	10

[1]Applicable state or local law may exceed this period.

7. DEVIATIONS, NONCONFORMANCES, AND ADVERSE EVENTS

⌗ **7.0 Deviations, Nonconformances, and Adverse Events**
The blood bank or transfusion service shall have policies, processes, and procedures to ensure the capture, assessment, investigation, and monitoring of deviations from or of failure to meet specified requirements. The investigation shall, when applicable, include an assessment of the effect of the deviation on donor eligibility and donor and patient safety. The responsibility for review and authority for the disposition of nonconforming blood, blood components, tissue, derivatives, critical materials, and services shall be defined. Deviations, nonconformances, and adverse events shall be reported in accordance with specified requirements and to outside agencies as required.*

⌗ **7.1 Nonconformances**
Upon discovery, nonconforming blood, blood components, tissue, derivatives, critical materials, and services shall be evaluated and their disposition determined.

7.1.1 Nonconforming blood, blood components, tissue, and derivatives shall be quarantined.

7.1.2 The unintended distribution or use of blood, blood components, tissue, derivatives, critical materials, or services that do not conform to specified requirements shall be prevented.

7.1.3 The blood bank or transfusion service shall have a process for:
1) The identification, quarantine, retrieval, and recall of nonconforming blood, blood components, tissue, and derivatives.
2) The identification and management of nonconforming services.
3) Notification of users, suppliers, and outside agencies as required.

⌗ **7.1.4 Released Nonconforming Blood, Blood Components, Tissue, or Derivatives**
Blood, blood components, tissue, or derivatives that are determined after release not to conform to specified requirements shall be evaluated to determine the effect of the nonconformance on the quality of the product. In cases where quality may have been affected, the non-

---

*21 CFR 606.171(b) and 21 CFR 1271.350.

conformance shall be reported to the customer. Records of the nature of nonconformances and subsequent actions taken, including acceptance for use, shall be maintained. Standard 9.1 applies.

7.1.4.1   Records shall include the disposition of the product or service, the rationale, and the name(s) of the individual(s) responsible for the decision.

7.2   Fatality Reporting
Fatalities confirmed to be caused by blood donation or blood transfusion shall be reported to outside agencies as required.[*]

7.3   Adverse Events Related to Donation
Adverse events related to the blood donation process shall be assessed, investigated, and monitored.

7.4   Adverse Events Related to Transfusion
There shall be a process for the administration of blood and blood components that includes the recognition, evaluation, and reporting of suspected transfusion-related adverse events. The medical director shall participate in the development of protocols used by the transfusing staff to identify, evaluate, and report adverse events related to transfusion. Standards 1.1.1 and 5.27 apply.

7.4.1   Recognition of and Response to Immediate Transfusion Reactions
There shall be processes and procedures for the transfusing staff for the recognition of and response to immediate transfusion reactions and for the recording of relevant information in the patient's medical record.

7.4.1.1   The process shall include:
1) Definition of signs and symptoms of suspected transfusion reactions.
2) Indications for interruption or discontinuation of the transfusion.
3) Evaluation and the timely clinical management of the patient.

7.4.1.2   When the transfusion is discontinued, the following shall be performed immediately:

---

[*]21 CFR 606.170(b).

1) The label on the blood containers and records shall be examined to detect errors in identifying the patient, blood, or blood component.
2) The blood bank or transfusion service and recipient's physician shall be notified. Signs and symptoms suggestive of mild allergic reactions (eg, urticaria) need not be reported to the blood bank or transfusion service.
3) The blood container (whether or not it contains any blood) shall be sent to the blood bank or transfusion service with, whenever possible, the attached transfusion set and intravenous solutions.
4) A posttransfusion sample shall be obtained from the patient and sent to the blood bank or transfusion service.

7.4.2 **Laboratory Evaluation and Reporting of Immediate Transfusion Reactions**
The blood bank or transfusion service shall have policies, processes, and procedures for the evaluation and reporting of suspected transfusion reactions, including prompt evaluation, review of clerical information by the blood bank or transfusion service, and notification of the blood bank or transfusion service medical director.

7.4.2.1 For suspected hemolytic transfusion reactions the evaluation shall include the following:
1) The patient's posttransfusion reaction serum or plasma shall be inspected for evidence of hemolysis. Pretransfusion samples shall be used for comparison.
2) A repeat ABO group determination shall be performed on the posttransfusion sample.
3) A direct antiglobulin test shall be performed on the posttransfusion sample. If the result is positive, the most recent pretransfusion sample shall be used for comparison.
4) The blood bank or transfusion service shall have a process for indicating under what circumstances additional testing shall be performed and what that testing shall be.
5) Review and interpretation by the medical director.

7.4.2.2 The blood bank or transfusion service shall have a process for evaluation for suspected nonhemolytic transfusion reactions including, but not limited to, febrile reactions, possible bacterial contamination, and TRALI.

7.4.2.3 Interpretation of the evaluation by the medical director shall be recorded in the patient's medical record and, if suggestive of hemolysis, bacterial contamination, TRALI, or other serious adverse event related to transfusion, the interpretation shall be reported to the patient's physician immediately. Standard 7.4.2.4 applies.

7.4.2.4 When a transfusion fatality or other serious, unexpected adverse event occurs that is suspected to be related to an attribute of a donor or a unit, the collecting facility shall be notified immediately and subsequently in writing.

7.4.3 Delayed Transfusion Reactions (Antigen-Antibody Reactions)
If a delayed transfusion reaction is suspected or detected, tests shall be performed to determine the cause. The results of the evaluation shall be reported to the patient's physician and recorded in the patient's medical record. Standard 7.4.2.4 applies.

7.4.4 Adverse Events Related to Tissue or Derivatives
The blood bank or transfusion service shall have a process for investigating adverse effects, disease transmission, or other suspected adverse events related to the use of tissue and derivatives and for promptly reporting such cases to the source facility, manufacturer, and outside agencies as required. Standards 7.4.5 and 7.4.6 apply.

7.4.5 Transmissible Diseases

7.4.5.1 Transfusion Service Reporting of Diseases Transmitted by Blood, Tissue, or Derivatives
The transfusion service shall have policies, processes, and procedures to evaluate and report diseases transmissible by blood, blood components, tissue, or derivatives. The policies, processes, and procedures shall include the following:

7.4.5.1.1 Prompt investigation of each event by the medical director.

7.4.5.1.2 If transmission is confirmed or not ruled out, the identity of the implicated blood, blood component(s), tissue, or derivative shall be reported to the collecting or source facility.

7.4.5.2 Collection Facility Investigation of Transmissible Diseases
The collection facility shall have policies, processes, and procedures for:
1) Investigating reports of diseases transmissible by blood, tissue, or derivatives.
2) Deferral of donors.
3) Communicating findings to the reporting facility.

7.4.6 Look-Back

7.4.6.1 Collection Facility
The collection facility shall have policies, processes, and procedures to notify consignees of blood or blood components from donors subsequently found to have, or be at risk for, relevant transmissible diseases.*

7.4.6.2 Transfusion Service
The transfusion service shall have policies, processes, and procedures to:

7.4.6.2.1 Identify recipients, if appropriate, of blood or blood components from donors subsequently found to have, or to be at risk for, relevant transmissible infections.

7.4.6.2.2 Notify, if appropriate, the recipient's physician and/or recipient as specified in FDA regulations and recommendations.†

---

*21 CFR 610.46-48 and 42 CFR 482.27(c).
FDA Guidance for Industry: Look back for Hepatitis C Virus (HCV): Product Quarantine, Consignee Notification, Further Testing, Product Disposition, and Notification of Transfusion Recipients Based on Donor Test Results Indicating Infection with HCV, August 24, 2007.
†21 CFR 610.46-48 and 42 CFR 482.27(c).
FDA Guidance for Industry: Lookback for Hepatitis C Virus (HCV): Product Quarantine, Consignee Notification, Further Testing, Product Disposition, and Notification of Transfusion Recipients Based on Donor Test Results Indicating Infection with HCV, August 24, 2007.

8. ASSESSMENTS: INTERNAL AND EXTERNAL

8.0 Assessments: Internal and External

The blood bank or transfusion service shall have policies, processes, and procedures to ensure that internal and external assessments of operations and quality systems are scheduled and conducted.

8.1 Management of Assessment Results

The results of internal and external assessments shall be reviewed by personnel having responsibility for the area being assessed.

8.1.1 When corrective action is taken, it shall be developed, implemented, and evaluated in accordance with Chapter 9, Process Improvement Through Corrective and Preventive Action.

8.1.2 The results of internal and external assessments and associated corrective and preventive actions shall be reviewed by executive management.

8.2 Monitoring

Transfusing facilities shall have a peer-review program that monitors and addresses transfusion practices for all categories of blood and blood components. The following shall be monitored:
1) Ordering practices.
2) Patient identification.
3) Sample collection and labeling.
4) Infectious and noninfectious adverse events.
5) Near-miss events.
6) Usage and discard.
7) Appropriateness of use.
8) Blood administration policies.
9) The ability of services to meet patient needs.
10) Compliance with peer-review recommendations.
11) Clinically relevant laboratory results.

Chapter 9, Process Improvement Through Corrective and Preventive Action, applies.

9. PROCESS IMPROVEMENT THROUGH CORRECTIVE AND PREVENTIVE ACTION

9.0 Process Improvement Through Corrective and Preventive Action

The blood bank or transfusion service shall have policies, processes, and procedures for data collection, analysis, and follow-up of issues requiring corrective and preventive action, including near-miss events.

9.1 Corrective Action

The blood bank or transfusion service shall have a process for corrective action of deviations, nonconformances, and complaints relating to blood, blood components, tissue, derivatives, critical materials, and services, which includes the following elements, as applicable:

1) Description of the event.
2) Investigation of the event.
3) Determination of the cause(s).
4) Implementation of the corrective action(s).
5) Evaluation to ensure that corrective action is taken and that it is effective.

9.2 Preventive Action

The blood bank or transfusion service shall have a process for preventive action that includes the following elements:

9.2.1 Review of information, including assessment results, proficiency testing results, quality control records, and complaints, to detect and analyze potential causes of nonconformances.

9.2.2 Determination of steps needed to respond to potential problems requiring preventive action.

9.2.3 Initiation of preventive action and application of controls to monitor effectiveness.

9.3 Quality Monitoring

The blood bank or transfusion service shall have a process to collect and evaluate quality indicator data on a scheduled basis.

10. FACILITIES AND SAFETY

10.0 Facilities and Safety

The blood bank or transfusion service shall have policies, processes, and procedures to ensure the provision of safe environmental conditions. The facility shall be suitable for the activities performed. Safety programs shall meet local, state, and federal regulations, where applicable. Standard 1.4 applies.

10.1 Safe Environment

The blood bank or transfusion service shall have processes to minimize and respond to environmentally related risks to the health and safety of employees, donors, volunteers, patients, and visitors. Suitable quarters, environment, and equipment shall be available to maintain safe operations.

10.2 Biological, Chemical, and Radiation Safety

The blood bank or transfusion service shall have a process for monitoring adherence to biological, chemical, and radiation safety standards and regulations, where applicable.

10.3 Discard of Blood, Components, Tissue, and Derivatives

Blood, blood components, tissue, and derivatives shall be handled and discarded in a manner that minimizes the potential for human exposure to infectious agents.

GLOSSARY

ABO Incompatibility Detection: Use of a method (eg, serologic or computer-based) to determine incompatibility of ABO group between donor and recipient.

Adverse Event: A complication in a donor or patient. Adverse events may occur in relation to a donation, a transfusion, or a diagnostic or therapeutic procedure.

Agreement: A contract, order, or understanding between two or more parties, such as between a facility and one of its customers.

Agreement Review: Systematic activities carried out before finalizing the agreement to ensure that requirements are adequately defined, free from ambiguity, documented, and achievable.

Allogeneic Donor: An individual from whom products intended for another person are collected.

Antibody Screen: A serologic method to detect the presence of clinically significant antibodies in recipients and/or donors.

Assessment: A systematic, independent examination that is performed at defined intervals and at sufficient frequency to determine whether actual activities comply with planned activities, are implemented effectively, and achieve objectives. Assessments usually include comparison of actual results to expected results. Types of assessments include external assessments, internal assessments, quality assessments, peer-review assessments, and self-assessments.

Autologous Donor: A person who acts as his or her own product donor.

Backup: Digital data storage media (magnetic tape, flash drive, CD, etc) containing copies of computer data.

Blood Bank: A facility that performs, or is responsible for the performance of, the collection, processing, storage, and/or distribution of human blood and/or blood components intended for transfusion and transplantation.

Blood Components: Products prepared from a whole blood collection or produced through an automated collection, eg, red cells, plasma, and platelets.

By a Method Known to: Use of published data to demonstrate the acceptability of a process or procedure, particularly for component preparation.

Certified by the Centers for Medicare and Medicaid Services (CMS): Having met the requirements of the Clinical Laboratory Improvement Amendments of 1988 for non-waived testing through inspection by the CMS, a deemed organization, or an exempt state agency.

Change Control: A structured method of revising a policy, process, or procedure, including hardware or software design, transition planning, and revisions to all related documents.

Clinically Significant Antibody: An antibody that is capable of causing shortened cell survival.

Closed System: A system, the contents of which are not exposed to air or outside elements during collection, preparation, and separation of components.

Collection Facility: A facility that collects blood and/or blood components from a donor.

Competence: Ability of an individual to perform a specific task according to procedures.

Compliance: See *Conformance*.

Conformance: Fulfillment of requirements. Requirements may be defined by customers, practice standards, regulatory agencies, or law.

Corrective Action: An activity performed to eliminate the cause of an existing nonconformance or other undesirable situation in order to prevent recurrence.

Critical Equipment/Materials/Tasks: A piece of equipment, material, service, or task that can affect the quality of the facility's products or services.

Crossmatch: A method (eg, serologic or computer-based) to detect incompatibility between donor and recipient.

Customer: The receiver of a product or service. A customer may be internal (eg, another department within the same organization) or external (eg, another organization).

Cytapheresis: A collection procedure where Whole Blood is removed and separated into components. One or more of the cellular components may be retained, while the remaining elements are combined and returned to the donor or patient.

Dedicated Donor: An individual who donates blood components intended for and used solely by a single identified recipient.

Derivatives: Sterile solutions of a specific protein(s) derived from blood or by recombinant technology (eg, albumin, plasma protein fraction, immune globulin, and factor concentrates).

Deviation: A departure from policies, processes, procedures, applicable regulations, standards, or specifications.

Disaster: An event (internal, local, or national) that can affect the safety and availability of the blood supply or the safety of staff, patients, volunteers, and donors.

Document (noun): Written or electronically generated information and work instructions. Examples of documents include quality manuals, procedures, or forms.

Document (verb): To capture information through writing or electronic media.

Equipment: A durable item, instrument, or device used in a process or procedure.

Event: A generic term used to encompass the terms "incident," "error," and "accident."

Executive Management: The highest level personnel within an organization, including employees and independent contractors, who have responsibility for the operations of the organization and who have the authority to establish or change the organization's quality policy. Executive management may be an individual or a group of individuals.

Expiration: The last day or time that the blood, blood component, tissue, derivative, or material(s) is considered suitable for use.

Facility: A location or operational area within an organization. The part of the organization that is assessed by the AABB and receives AABB accreditation for its specific activities.

Final Inspection: To measure, examine, or test one or more characteristics of a unit of blood or a blood component, a tissue, or a service and compare results with specified requirements in order to establish whether conformance is achieved before distribution or issue.

Guidelines: Documented recommendations.

Indefinite Deferral: A deferral applied to a donor who is not eligible to donate blood for someone else for an unspecified period of time.

Inspect: To measure, examine, or test one or more characteristics of a product or service and compare results with specific requirements.

Irradiated: Exposure of blood components to x-rays or gamma rays at a minimum dose of 25 Gy (2500 cGy) targeted to the central portion of the irradiation canister or irradiation field to prevent the proliferation of T lymphocytes.

ISBT 128: A standard for the identification, terminology, coding, and labeling for blood, cellular therapy, and tissue products. When linear bar codes are used, Code 128 symbology is utilized.

Issue: To release for clinical use (transfusion or transplantation).

Label: An inscription affixed to a unit of blood or a blood component, a tissue, a derivative, or a sample for identification.

Labeling: Information that is required or selected to accompany a unit of blood or a blood component, a tissue, a derivative, or a sample, which may include content, identification, description of processes, storage requirements, expiration date, cautionary statements, or indications for use.

Lived with: Resided in the same dwelling (eg, home, dormitory room, or apartment).

Maintain: To keep in the current state.

Master List of Documents: A reference list, record, or repository of a facility's policies, processes, procedures, forms, and labels related to the standards that includes information for document control.

Material: A good or supply item used in the manufacturing process. Materials are a type of input product. Reagents are a type of material.

Near-Miss Event: An unexpected occurrence that did not adversely affect the outcome but could have resulted in a serious adverse event.

Neonate: A child less than 4 months of age.

Nonconformance: Failure to meet requirements.

Open System: A system, the contents of which are exposed to air and outside elements during preparation and separation of components.

Organization: An institution, or part thereof, that has its own functions and executive management.

Permanent Deferral: A deferral applied to a donor who will never be eligible to donate blood for someone else.

Policy: A documented general principle that guides present and future decisions.

Preventive Action: An action taken to reduce the potential for nonconformances or other undesirable situations.

Procedure: A series of tasks usually performed by one person according to instructions.

Process: A set of related tasks and activities that accomplish a work goal.

Process Control: The efforts to standardize and control processes in order to produce predictable output.

Product: A tangible result of a process or procedure.

Proficiency Testing: The structured evaluation of laboratory methods that assesses the suitability of processes, procedures, equipment, materials, and personnel.

Qualification: With respect to individuals, the aspects of an individual's education, training, and experience that are necessary to successfully meet the requirements of a position. Specifically for equipment, verification that specified attributes required to accomplish the desired task have been met.

Quality: Characteristics of a unit of blood or a blood component, a tissue, a derivative, a sample, a critical material, or a service that bear on its ability to meet requirements, including those defined during agreement review.

Quality Control: Testing routinely performed on materials and equipment to ensure their proper function.

Quality Indicator Data: Information that may be collected and used to determine whether an organization is meeting its quality objectives as defined by top management in its quality policy. Indicators are measured by data for movement or regression with regard to those quality intentions. The data used for monitoring a quality indicator may consist of single-source data or multiple-source data, as long as it is clear how the data will come together to define the indicator.

Quality System: The organizational structure, responsibilities, policies, processes, procedures, and resources established by executive management to achieve quality.

Quarantine: To isolate nonconforming blood, blood components, tissue, derivatives, or materials to prevent their distribution or use.

Reagent: A substance used to perform an analytical procedure. A substance used (as in detecting or measuring a component or preparing a product) because of its biological or chemical activity.

Record (noun): Information captured in writing or through electronically generated media that provides objective evidence of activities that have been performed or results that have been achieved, such as test records or audit results. Records do not exist until the activity has been performed and documented.

Record (verb): To capture information for use in records through writing or electronic media.

Reference Standards: Specified requirements defined by the AABB (see *Specified Requirements*). Reference standards define how or within what parameters an activity shall be performed and are more detailed than quality system requirements.

Regulations: Rules promulgated by federal, state, or local authorities to implement laws enacted by legislative bodies.

Release: Removal of product from quarantine or in-process status for distribution.

Segregate: To separate or isolate products by a method known to clearly identify them and to minimize the possibility of their unintended distribution or use.

Service: An intangible result of a process or procedure.

Sexual Contact: Any of the following activities (whether or not a condom or other protection was used): vaginal sex (contact between penis and vagina); oral sex (contact between mouth or tongue and vagina, penis, or anus); or anal sex (contact between penis and anus).

Shall: A term used to indicate a requirement.

Special Transfusion Requirements: Refers to a patient's medical need for components that have been modified, such as components that are irradiated, washed, or leukocyte reduced; components from special sources, such as autologous or directed sources; components that need special handling (eg, being subjected to the heat of a blood warming device); or components that contain special attributes (eg, CMV-seronegative or antigen-negative).

Specified Requirements: Any requirements in these *BBTS Standards*, including, but not limited to, FDA requirements; requirements of a facility's internal policies, processes, and procedures; manufacturers' instructions; customer agreements; practice standards; and requirements of accrediting organizations such as the AABB.

Supplier: An entity that provides an input material or service.

Supplier Qualification: An evaluation method designed to ensure that input materials and services (eg, materials, blood, blood components, tissue, derivatives, patient blood samples) obtained from a supplier meet specified requirements.

Temporary Deferral: A deferral placed on a donor who is not eligible to donate for a specified period of time.

Tissue: A group of functional cells and/or intercellular matrix intended for implantation, transplantation, or other therapy (eg, cornea, ligaments, bone). Cellular therapy products covered by the AABB's *Standards for Cellular Therapy Services* are not included herein. A cellular therapy product is defined by the 6th edition of *Standards for Cellular Therapy Services* as somatic cell-based products (eg, mobilized hematopoietic progenitor cells, cord blood, pancreatic islets) that are procured from a donor and intended for manipulation and/or administration.

Traceability: The ability to follow the history of a product or service by means of recorded identification.

Transfusion-Related Acute Lung Injury (TRALI): A new acute lung injury (ALI) within 6 hours of a completed transfusion.

Transfusion Service: A facility that performs one or more of the following activities:

compatibility testing, storage, selection, and issuing of blood and blood components to intended recipients. Transfusion services do not routinely collect blood or process Whole Blood into components (except Red Blood Cells and Recovered Plasma).

Transmissible Disease: A disease or condition caused by a virus, bacteria, fungus, parasite, or agent of transmissible spongiform encephalopathy that may be transmitted by transfusion of blood or blood components or by tissue implantation or transplantation or administration of derivatives.

True Positive: A positive result on both the initial test and the confirmatory test. Specifically for bacteria detection, a confirmatory test is a culture-based test performed on a different sample than the blood culture bottle or other sample used for the initial test. For example, a sample source for the confirmatory test could be the original platelet component. A subculture of the initial positive culture is not an adequate sample for this purpose. If initial testing was culture-based, the confirmatory test can use the same method applied to the alternate sample source.

Unit: A container of blood or one of its components in a suitable volume of anticoagulant obtained from a collection of blood from one donor.

Urticaria Reaction: The development of hives, maculopapular rash, or similar allergic manifestation.

User-Defined Tables: Tables containing data used by computer programs to direct their operations. Typically, user-defined tables contain data that are unique to a specific installation and may change from system to system.

Validation: Establishing recorded evidence that provides a high degree of assurance that a specific process will consistently produce an outcome meeting its predetermined specifications and quality attributes.

Verification: Confirmation by examination and provision of objective evidence that specified requirements have been met.

"CROSSWALK" BETWEEN THE 28th AND 29th EDITIONS OF STANDARDS

The following "crosswalk" traces each standard in the 28th and 29th editions of *Standards for Blood Banks and Transfusion Services*. Each standard in the 29th edition corresponds with its predecessor in the 28th edition. Standards in the 29th edition appearing in bold are new or have been changed. The "crosswalk" is offered as assistance to those who will be updating their facility's procedures to be compliant with the most current edition of *BBTS Standards*. Its use should not take place of a thorough, line-by-line analysis of each standard.

29th	28th	29th	28th
1.0	1.0	3.3	3.3
1.1	1.1	3.4	3.4
1.1.1	1.1.1	3.5	3.5
1.2	1.2	**3.5.1**	3.5.1
1.2.1	1.2.1	3.5.1.1	3.5.1.1
1.2.2	1.2.2	3.5.1.2	3.5.1.2
1.3	1.3	3.5.2	3.5.2
1.3.1	1.3.1	3.6	3.6
1.3.2	1.3.2	3.6.1	3.6.1
1.4	1.4	**3.6.2**	3.6.2
1.4.1	1.4.1	3.6.3	3.6.3
1.5	1.5	3.7	3.7
1.6	1.6	3.7.1	3.7.1
2.0	2.0	3.7.2	3.7.2
2.1	2.1	3.7.3	3.7.3
2.1.1	2.1.1	3.8	3.8
2.1.2	2.1.2	3.9	3.9
2.1.3	2.1.3	3.9.1	3.9.1
2.1.3.1	2.1.3.1	3.9.2	3.9.2
2.1.4	2.1.4	3.9.3	3.9.3
2.1.4.1	2.1.4.1	3.9.4	3.9.4
3.0	3.0	3.9.5	3.9.5
3.1	3.1	4.0	4.0
3.2	3.2	4.1	4.1
3.2.1	3.2.1	4.1.1	4.1.1
3.2.2	3.2.2	4.1.2	4.1.2
3.2.3	3.2.3, 3.2.3.1	4.1.2.1	4.1.2.1

Crosswalk

29th	28th	29th	28th
4.2	4.2	**5.1.8.1.3**	5.1.8.1.3
4.2.1	4.2.1	5.1.8.1.3.1	5.1.8.1.3.1
4.2.2	4.2.2	5.1.8.1.4	5.1.8.1.4
4.3	4.3	5.1.8.2	5.1.8.2
4.3.1	4.3.1	5.1.8.2.1	5.1.8.2.1
4.3.2	4.3.2	5.2	5.2
4.3.2.1	4.3.2.1	5.2.1, #1	5.2.1, #1
5.0	5.0	5.2.1, #2	5.2.1, #2
5.1	5.1	5.2.1, #3	5.2.1, #3
5.1.1	5.1.1	**5.2.1, #4**	5.2.3.1
5.1.2	5.1.2	5.2.1, #5	5.2.1, #4
5.1.3	5.1.3	5.2.1, #6	5.2.1, #5
5.1.3.1	5.1.3.2	5.2.2	5.2.2
5.1.3.2	5.1.3.1	5.2.3	5.2.3
5.1.4	5.1.4	5.2.4	5.2.4
5.1.4.1	5.1.4.1	5.3	5.3
5.1.5	5.1.5	5.3.1	5.3.1
5.1.5.1	5.1.5.1	5.3.2	5.3.2
5.1.5.1.1	5.1.5.1.1	5.3.2.1	5.3.2.1
5.1.5.2	5.1.5.2	5.3.3	5.3.3
5.1.6	5.1.6	5.3.3.1	5.3.3.1
5.1.6.1	5.1.6.1	5.3.3.2	5.3.3.2
5.1.6.2	5.1.6.2	5.3.4	5.3.4
5.1.6.3	5.1.6.3	5.3.4.1	5.3.4.1
5.1.6.3.1, #1	5.1.6.3.1, #1	5.4	5.4
5.1.6.3.1, #2	5.1.6.3.1, #2	5.4.1	5.4.1
5.1.6.3.1, #3	5.1.6.3.1, #3	5.4.1.1	5.4.4.1
5.1.6.3.1, #4	5.1.6.3.1, #4	**5.4.1.2**	**New**
5.1.6.3.1, #5	5.1.6.3.1, #5	5.4.2	5.4.2
5.1.6.3.1, #6	5.1.6.3.1, #6	**5.4.2.1**	**New**
5.1.6.4	5.1.6.4	5.4.3	5.4.3
5.1.6.5	5.1.6.5	5.4.3.1	5.4.3.1
5.1.6.5.1	5.1.6.5.1	5.4.3.2	5.4.3.2
5.1.6.5.2	5.1.6.5.2	5.4.4	5.4.4
5.1.6.5.3	5.1.6.5.3	5.4.4.1	5.4.4.1
5.1.7	5.1.7	5.4.4.2	5.4.4.2
5.1.8	5.1.8	5.4.4.3	5.4.4.3
5.1.8.1	5.1.8.1	5.4.4.4	5.4.4.4
5.1.8.1.1	5.1.8.1.1	5.4.4.5	5.4.4.5
5.1.8.1.2	5.1.8.1.2	5.5	5.5

29th	28th
5.5.1	5.5.1
5.5.2	5.5.2
5.5.2.1	5.5.2.1
5.5.2.2	5.5.2.2
5.5.2.2.1	5.5.2.2.1
5.5.3	5.5.3
5.5.3.1	5.5.3.1
5.5.3.2	5.5.3.2
5.5.3.3	5.5.3.3
5.5.3.4	5.5.3.4
5.5.3.4.1	5.5.3.4.1
5.5.3.4.2	5.5.3.4.2
5.5.3.4.3	5.5.3.4.3
5.5.3.5	5.5.3.5
5.5.3.5.1	5.5.3.5.1
5.5.3.5.2	5.5.3.5.2
5.5.4	5.5.4
5.6	5.6
5.6.1	5.6.1
5.6.2	5.6.2
5.6.2.1	5.6.2.1
5.6.3	5.6.3
5.6.3.1	5.6.3.1
5.6.3.1.1	5.6.3.1.1
5.6.3.2	5.6.3.2
5.6.3.3	5.6.3.3
5.6.4	5.6.4
5.6.5	5.6.5
5.6.5.1	5.6.5.1
5.6.6	5.6.6
5.6.6.1	5.6.6.1
5.6.6.2	5.6.6.2
5.6.6.2.1	5.6.6.2.1
5.6.7	5.6.7
5.6.7.1	5.6.7.1
5.7	5.7
5.7.1	5.7.1
5.7.2	5.7.2
5.7.2.1	5.7.2.1
5.7.2.1.1	5.7.2.1.1

29th	28th
5.7.2.1.2	5.7.2.1.2
5.7.3	5.7.4
5.7.3.1	5.7.4.1
5.7.3.2	5.7.4.2
5.7.3.2.1	5.7.4.2.1
5.7.3.3	5.7.4.3.3
5.7.4	5.7.5
5.7.4.1	5.7.5.1
5.7.4.1.1	5.7.5.1.1
5.7.4.2	5.7.5.2
5.7.4.2.1	5.7.5.2.1
5.7.4.3	5.7.5.3
5.7.4.4	5.7.5.4
5.7.4.5	5.7.5.5
5.7.4.6	5.7.5.6
5.7.4.7	5.7.5.7
5.7.4.8	5.7.5.8
5.7.4.8.1	5.7.5.8.1
5.7.4.9	5.7.5.9
5.7.4.9.1	5.7.5.9.1
5.7.4.10	5.7.5.10
5.7.4.10.1	5.7.5.10.1
5.7.4.11	**New**
5.7.4.12	5.7.5.11
5.7.4.13	5.7.5.12
5.7.4.14	5.7.5.13
5.7.4.15	5.7.5.14
5.7.4.16	5.7.5.15
5.7.4.17	5.7.5.16
5.7.4.18	5.7.5.17
5.7.4.19	5.7.5.18
5.7.4.20	5.7.5.19
5.7.4.21	5.7.5.20
5.7.4.22	5.7.5.21
5.7.4.23	**New**
5.7.4.24	5.7.5.22
5.8	5.8
5.8.1	5.8.1
5.8.2	5.8.2
5.8.3	5.8.3

29th	28th	29th	28th
5.8.3.1	5.8.3.1	5.14.5	5.13.5
5.8.3.2	5.8.3.2	5.15	5.14
5.8.3.3	5.8.3.3	5.15.1	5.14.1
5.8.4	**New**	5.15.2	5.14.2
5.8.5	5.8.4	5.15.2.1	5.14.2.1
5.8.5.1	5.8.4.1	5.15.3	5.14.3
5.8.5.2	5.8.4.2	5.15.4	5.14.4
5.8.6	5.8.5	5.15.5	5.14.5
5.8.6.1	5.8.5.1	5.16	5.15
5.8.7	5.8.6	5.16.1	5.15.1
5.9	5.9	5.16.1.1	5.15.1.1
5.9.1	5.9.1	**5.16.2**	5.15.2
5.9.2	5.9.2	5.16.2.1	5.15.2.1
5.9.3	5.9.3	**5.16.2.2**	5.15.2.2
5.9.4	5.9.4	5.16.2.3	5.15.2.3
5.9.5	5.9.5	5.16.2.4	5.15.2.4
5.9.5.1	5.9.5.1	5.16.2.5	5.15.2.5
5.9.5.2	5.9.5.2	5.17	5.16
5.10	5.10	5.17.1	5.16.1
5.11	5.11	5.17.1.1	5.16.1.1
5.11.1	5.11.1	5.17.1.2	5.16.1.2
5.11.1.1	5.11.1.1	5.17.1.3	5.16.1.3
5.11.2	5.11.2	5.17.2	5.16.2
5.11.2.1	5.11.2.1	5.17.2.1	5.16.2.1
5.11.2.2	5.11.2.2	5.17.2.2	5.16.2.2
5.11.2.3	5.11.2.3	**5.18**	**New**
5.11.3	5.11.3	5.19	5.17
5.11.4	5.11.4	5.19.1	5.17.1
5.12	5.12	5.19.2	5.17.2
5.12.1	5.12.1	5.19.3	5.17.3
5.13	**New**	5.19.3.1	5.17.3.1
5.14	5.13	5.19.3.1.1	5.17.3.1.1
5.14.1	5.13.1	5.19.3.1.2	5.17.3.1.2
5.14.2	5.13.2	5.19.3.1.3	5.17.3.1.3
5.14.3	5.13.3	5.19.4	5.17.4
5.14.3.1	5.13.3.1	5.19.5	5.17.5
5.14.3.2	5.13.3.2	**5.19.6**	**New**
5.14.3.3	5.13.3.3	5.20	5.18
5.14.3.4	5.13.3.4	5.21	5.19
5.14.4	5.13.4	5.22	5.20

29th	28th	29th	28th
5.22.1	5.20.1	**5.1.8A**	5.1.8A
5.23	5.21	**5.4.1A**	5.4.1A
5.24, #1	5.22, #1	6.0	6.0
5.24, #2	5.22, #2	6.1	6.1
5.24, #3	5.22, #3	6.1.1	6.1.1
5.24, #4	5.22, #4	6.1.2	6.1.2
5.24, #5	5.22, #5	6.1.3	6.1.3
5.24, #6	5.22, #6	6.1.4	6.1.4
5.25	5.23	6.1.5	6.1.5
5.26	5.24	6.1.6	6.1.6
5.27	5.25	6.1.7	6.1.7
5.27.1	5.25.1	6.2	6.2
5.27.2	5.25.2	6.2.1	6.2.1
5.27.3	5.25.3	6.2.1.1	6.2.1.1
5.27.4	5.25.4	6.2.1.2	6.2.1.2
5.27.5	5.25.5	6.2.2	6.2.2
5.27.5.1	5.25.5.1	6.2.3	6.2.3
5.28	5.26	6.2.4, #1	6.2.3.1, #1
5.28.1	5.26.1	6.2.4, #2	6.2.3.1, #2
5.28.1.1	5.26.1.1	6.2.4, #3	6.2.3.1, #3
5.28.2	5.26.2	6.2.4, #4	6.2.3.1, #4
5.28.3	5.26.3	**6.2.4, #5**	6.2.3.1, #5
5.28.4	5.26.4	6.2.4, #6	6.2.3.1, #6
5.28.5	5.26.5	6.2.4, #7	6.2.3.1, #7
5.28.6	5.26.6	6.2.4, #8	6.2.3.1, #8
5.28.7	5.26.7	6.2.4.1	6.2.3.2
5.28.8	5.26.8	6.2.5	6.2.4
5.28.9	5.26.9	6.2.5.1	6.2.4.1
5.28.10	5.26.10	6.2.6	6.2.5
5.29	5.27	6.2.6.1	6.2.5.1
5.29.1	5.27.1	6.2.6.2	6.2.5.2
5.29.2	5.27.2	6.2.6.3	6.2.5.3
5.29.3	5.27.3	6.2.7	6.2.6
5.30	5.28	6.2.7.1	6.2.6.1
5.30.1	5.28.1	6.2.7.1.1	6.2.6.1.1
5.30.2	5.28.2	6.2.7.1.2	6.2.6.1.2
5.30.3	5.28.3	6.2.8	6.2.7
5.30.4	5.28.4	6.2.9	6.2.8
5.30.5	5.28.5	6.2A	6.2A
5.1.6A	5.1.6A	**6.2B**	6.2B

Crosswalk

29th	28th	29th	28th
6.2C	6.2C	7.4.6.2.1	7.4.6.2.1
6.2D	6.2D	7.4.6.2.2	7.4.6.2.2
6.2E	6.2E	8.0	8.0
7.0	7.0	8.1	8.1
7.1	7.1	8.1.1	8.1.1
7.1.1	7.1.1	8.1.2	8.1.2
7.1.2	7.1.2	8.2, #1	8.2, #1
7.1.3	7.1.3	8.2, #2	8.2, #2
7.1.4	7.1.4	8.2, #3	8.2, #3
7.1.4.1	7.1.4.1	8.2, #4	8.2, #4
7.2	7.2	8.2, #5	8.2, #5
7.3	7.3	8.2, #6	8.2, #6
7.4	7.4	8.2, #7	8.2, #7
7.4.1	7.4.1	8.2, #8	8.2, #8
7.4.1.1	7.4.1.1	8.2, #9	8.2, #9
7.4.1.2	7.4.1.2	8.2, #10	8.2, #10
7.4.2	7.4.2	**8.2, #11**	8.2, #11
7.4.2.1	7.4.2.1	9.0	9.0
7.4.2.2	7.4.2.2	9.1, #1	9.1, #1
7.4.2.3	7.4.2.3	9.1, #2	9.1, #2
7.4.2.4	7.4.2.4	9.1, #3	9.1, #3
7.4.3	7.4.3	**9.1, #4**	**New**
7.4.4	7.4.4	9.1, #5	9.1, #4
7.4.5	7.4.5	9.2	9.2
7.4.5.1	7.4.5.1	9.2.1	9.2.1
7.4.5.1.1	7.4.5.1.1	9.2.2	9.2.2
7.4.5.1.2	7.4.5.1.2	9.2.3	9.2.3
7.4.5.2	7.4.5.2	9.3	9.3
7.4.6	7.4.6	10.0	10.0
7.4.6.1	7.4.6.1	10.1	10.1
7.4.6.2	7.4.6.2	10.2	10.2
		10.3	10.3

INDEX

Index

Index

Index